Herbal and Magical Medicine

Herbal and Magical Medicine

Traditional Healing Today

Edited by James Kirkland, Holly F. Mathews,

C. W. Sullivan III, and Karen Baldwin

DUKE UNIVERSITY PRESS *Durham & London, 1992*

Third printing, 1997

Library of Congress Cataloging-in-Publication Data
appear on the last printed page of this book.

For Paula, Becky, and Craig
—James Kirkland

For my husband and colleague, Ronald Hoag, with grateful appreciation for his assistance with and support for this project—Holly Mathews

For Barre, Bill, Bob, Dick, Ed, Jack, Linda, Neil, Polly, Sharon, Sue, Susan, Suzi, Twilo, and Tom—the Oregon folklore gang (1971–1977)
—C. W. Sullivan III

For Polly Stewart and Ernest Marshall—my best friends and great supporters of this work—and to the memory of Professor Wayland Debs Hand, whose scholarship is fundamental for the study of folk medicine and belief, internationally and in North Carolina
—Karen Baldwin

Contents

Preface

Karen Baldwin

Herbal and Magical Medicine: Traditional Healing Today is a collaboration among scholars and specialists in folklore, anthropology, clinical medicine, psychiatry, and ethnobotany to produce a volume whose focus is the contemporary, widely spread, and culturally significant systems of health and medical belief and practice variously known as "folk," "vernacular," or "alternative" medicine. "Traditional" and "folk" are the terms used interchangeably throughout this book to designate any medical concept or behavior based on noninstitutionalized oral traditional processes rather than on formal academic and clinical training.

The book demonstrates, within one region, how folk medical systems operate in tandem and conjunction with scientific biomedicine, how the folk medical systems of culturally differentiated groups converge and influence each other, and how folk medical ideas and practices are integral to individual patients' expressions of kin and community-based cultural identity.

Traditional healing has long been the subject of scholarly study by folklorists at East Carolina University (ECU), where the English Department's undergraduate American Folklore course attracts several hundred students a year and the ECU Folklore Archive holds one of the largest university-based, regional collections of individual genre items and contextual studies in the country. The potential for multidisciplinary studies became apparent in the spring of 1979 when James Kirkland and Karen Baldwin, then working with archive and field research in folk medicine, learned of the video documentation of a nearby herbalist healer, Emma Dupree, by Walter Shepherd of the ECU School of Medicine and the late

James Young, until his death a medical anthropologist in the Department of Sociology and Anthropology. Shepherd was eager to begin collaborative studies of patient-practitioner relationships, health and illness behaviors in community settings, and other promising subjects.

Agreeing that they should concentrate initially on developing the research potential of the folk medical holdings in the ECU Folklore Archive, the three worked out a plan that almost immediately produced significant results: the School of Medicine funded a position for a research assistant to work with Baldwin, the archive director, culling folk medical materials from the more than 100,000 individually recorded items and 5,000 full-context manuscript collections in the archive. Baldwin indexed and annotated these materials according to volume 6 of *The Frank C. Brown Collection of North Carolina Folklore,* and worked with colleague John Warren, who designed programs for computer-assisted humanities research, to develop an information retrieval system. The English Department added to the School of Medicine support by assigning two graduate assistants to the project and the University Research Committee awarded professors Kirkland and Baldwin a grant to conduct a survey of representative healers and patients identified in the archive search.

Wishing to expand and develop interdisciplinary cooperation, Baldwin and Kirkland next organized a panel of papers for the annual meeting of the American Folklore Society (AFS). Baldwin chaired the panel, Kirkland read an earlier version of the essay included here, and they invited participation from others whose papers were revised for inclusion here: C. W. Sullivan III, another folklorist at ECU; David J. Hufford, an authority on alternative health care systems and a member of the Behavioral Sciences faculty at the Hershey Medical Center of Pennsylvania State University; and Robert Sammons, then a faculty member of the ECU Psychology Department and a practicing hypnotherapist. The AFS panel combined theoretical discussions of the nature and functions of folk medicine in contemporary life with pragmatic studies of pregnancy and childbirth beliefs, magico-religious healing practices, and the relationship between folk healers and professionally trained hypnotherapists.

Encouraged by the responsiveness of the AFS audience and by the support offered by one of its most prominent members, Professor Wayland Hand, Kirkland and Baldwin began disseminating information about their research and planning for this volume of interrelated studies. Through the ECU Medical Humanities Committee, they established contacts with two other authorities—Holly F. Mathews, a medical anthropologist, and Peter R. Lichstein, a specialist in internal medicine—both of whom had been doing research on rootworking and provided complementary articles on the subject. Professor Hand, too, agreed to contribute an introductory essay for the volume and, up until the time of his death, had read and written initial comments for most of the studies in the collection.

Professors Sullivan and Mathews agreed to share the work of editing the volume and three final articles were contributed by scholars outside ECU: Edward M. Croom, an expert on the ethnobotany of the Lumbee Indians; Linda Camino, Research Assistant Professor of Anthropology at George Washington University and an authority on the religious concept of spiritual heart trouble; and Richard Blaustein, Director of the Center for Appalachian Culture and Services at East Tennessee State University, whose theoretical essay introduces the body of interrelated studies.

Treating a variety of topics and using a variety of analytical approaches, the contributors to this volume all emphasize the importance, indeed, oftentimes, the *primacy* of traditional folk medicine for individuals in communities. Each scholar/specialist also contributes to the multidisciplinary description of people throughout the eastern regions of North Carolina and Virginia who are vitally involved with kin and community-based folk traditional medical systems, people whose active folk medical traditions are similar to contemporary practices among other groups in other regions of the country.

Working on this volume has been an exciting process, and there are many people to thank for their contributions, besides those already mentioned, the authors, and their informants. Bobbie Houston and Janet Whitehurst did the initial archive research and Whitehurst also transcribed fieldwork tape recordings. Teresa Stallings, Keith Stallings, Judy Bowers, Monica Konarski-Tischler, Robin Whaley, Resa Crane-Roger, David McKeel, and Carol Thompson all worked with compiling and checking the accuracy of the bibliography. Robin Whaley and Resa Crane-Roger typed the bibliography. Donna Evans, Tina Moore, Robbin Nelson, and Patsy Collier all typed portions of the manuscript and provided other secretarial assistance. Joel Huddleston, Robin Cox, Steve Daughtridge, Dexter Hill, and Helene Woodard, former ECU folklore students, provided contacts with folk medicine informants.

Introduction: A Regional Approach and Multidisciplinary Perspective

Holly F. Mathews

This volume of essays documents the contemporary practice of several widespread and culturally significant systems of "traditional" or "folk" medicine in the eastern regions of North Carolina and Virginia. Traditional and folk are terms used interchangeably throughout this book to refer to "those beliefs and practices relating to disease which are the products of indigenous cultural development and are not explicitly derived from the conceptual framework of modern medicine" (Hughes 151). Such indigenous medical systems are known by a confusing plethora of terms including alternative, unorthodox, vernacular, fringe, nontraditional, unofficial, and ethnomedical. The labeling of these systems as "traditional" is consistent with the terminology embraced by the World Health Organization (WHO) during their International Conference on Primary Health Care in 1978 (Mahler 7). WHO officials emphasize that traditional medicines are found in all societies throughout all periods of history and predate the rise of modern scientific medicine or allopathy at the beginning of the nineteenth century (Bannerman et al. 9–11).

Any culture's traditional medicine includes perceptions of health and definitions of illness, beliefs about etiology and appropriate preventive and curative practices, as well as roles for indigenous practitioners who not only treat illness but also act to restore health for individuals and a sense of well-being to the community as a whole. Traditional beliefs and practices do not develop in isolation but are part of an integrated set of social institutions within a cultural system. Consequently, they serve many functions for adherents and are often highly resistant to change even when the cultural tradition itself is no longer viable.

In many parts of the world, the expansion of Western culture has brought scientific biomedicine into direct confrontation with traditional care. Yet both here and abroad, adherents of traditional medicine do not necessarily embrace all aspects of the scientific system when it becomes available to them. The study of how and why traditional beliefs and practices persist in the wake of such change is of vital importance for those who want to improve the health status of a population. A key goal of the authors in this volume is to describe and explain the logic of traditional medical systems to health planners and practitioners in order to suggest how they can be integrated more effectively with biomedicine in order to improve the overall delivery of care.

More useful than a collection of individualized studies done in disparate and culturally disconnected regions of the United States, this book applies a multidisciplinary approach to a coherent cultural center of traditional folk medical systems as practiced by Native, Anglo-, and African-Americans in the eastern regions of North Carolina and Virginia. This book is unique because it carefully documents the traditional medicines of a long-settled and culturally important region that has received little serious scholarly attention; it is also important because it articulates a model of multidisciplinary inquiry applicable to the study of traditional medicine in any cultural context.

The eastern region of Virginia and North Carolina was among the first areas of the United States to be permanently colonized by the British. Inhabited by a thriving population of Native Americans at the time of contact, it remains home today to the largest number of Indians found east of the Mississippi River. In addition, a vibrant African-American culture has endured and flourished since the earliest days of slavery in the colony. Surprisingly, however, the existence of these diverse cultural traditions in a region relatively unaltered by outside influences has not occasioned much systematic scholarly inquiry. Most folklore research in the two states has been done in the Appalachian zone while the well-known and prestigious Frank C. Brown collection of North Carolina folklore was drawn almost exclusively from the piedmont region.

The coexistence of these three traditions, however, presents researchers from different disciplines with the unprecedented opportunity to study the ways in which folk medical systems of culturally differentiated groups converge and influence one another, operate in tandem and conjunction with scientific biomedicine, and provide beliefs and practices integral to the individual's expressions of kin and community-based identity. While each of these groups maintained its own unique medical tradition, culture contact led to the diffusion of certain beliefs and practices across system boundaries; the expansion and eventual dominance of Christianity has given each a common theological underpinning. Significantly, these beliefs and practices persist and remain strong, providing adherents with a continuity of tradition that influences and shapes their encounters with the ever-expanding biomedical system. A brief description of the history and present sociodemographic profile of the region illustrates some of the reasons why these traditions have endured.

The eastern region of Virginia and North Carolina lies within the broad coastal plain that extends from the Atlantic Ocean on the east to the fall line of the major rivers in the piedmont zone to the west. The tidewater zone itself extends inland from the coast as far as the effects of the tide are visible and encompasses many of the region's major coastal port cities including Norfolk and Newport News in Virginia; and Washington, New Bern, Jacksonville, and Wilmington in North Carolina. The geographic diversity of the region is striking. The tidewater zone is low and swampy with numerous bays, inlets, and natural lakes. To the west, the coastal plain contains much fertile farmland and a zone of pine-covered dunes in southeastern North Carolina (see Merrens 32–49, for a more detailed description of the land).

The eastern regions were first explored by the French and Spanish. It was the English, however, under the leadership of Sir Walter Raleigh, who attempted to establish the first colony in the area on Roanoke Island, part of the Outer Banks of North Carolina. This attempt failed, and the first permanent settlement in the east was the English colony at Jamestown, Virginia, established in 1607. Large-scale colonization in eastern North Carolina began in the 1650s as Virginians moved south in search of good farmland (Lefler and Powell 31–35). Settlers, primarily of English and European backgrounds, eventually followed from other colonies; but then as now, few of these inhabitants were foreign born (Lefler 423). The early settlers were primarily agriculturalists, and many depended on imported slave labor to operate the plantation economy based on the cultivation of cotton and tobacco. African-American slaves accounted for about one-third of the population of the region at the time of emancipation and today African Americans comprise approximately 22 percent of the population (Lefler 423).

When the first colonists arrived, they encountered an estimated 25,000 Native Americans living in highly stratified, agriculturally based chiefdoms in the eastern zone (Wetmore 49). As white settlement expanded, conflicts with the Indians increased, culminating in a long series of skirmishes in the region that began in 1675 with the Susquehanna War in Virginia (Rights 34) and ended with the Tuscarora Wars in eastern North Carolina, fought between 1711 and 1713 (Lefler and Powell 66–74). The cumulative effects of disease, slavery, the disruption of agriculture and hunting by the encroachment of whites, and deaths in warfare reduced the Indian population to just over 1,000 by the 1730s (Merrens 20). The surviving Tuscarora either fled to New York State or moved onto reservation land in eastern North Carolina, while the few remaining members of the other tribes banded together and retreated into the more rural and isolated parts of the region (Wetmore 40). Of necessity, most of these Indians intermarried with whites and blacks, adopted the language of English and the customs of the colonists, and, in the process, lost most of their distinctive Indian heritage. Today their descendants are located primarily in eastern North Carolina and identify themselves as either Tuscarora, Haliwa, Coharie, Waccamaw-Siouans, or Lumbee (Wetmore 170–71). None of these groups has been granted federal recognition, primarily because of the difficulty each has in proving a continuous cultural and linguistic tradition. Nonetheless, they are the largest group of Native Americans located east of the Mississippi River, and the Lumbee, who numbered 35,400 in the 1980 census, are the largest tribal group in the state of North Carolina (U.S. Department of Commerce).

The disruption caused by the Indian wars along with the relative isolation resulting from a lack of transportation networks led to slow growth for the eastern region during the 1700s. In North Carolina, for example, the government of the state was dominated by the landed aristocracy of the east and, after the Revolutionary War, economic decline caused thousands of inhabitants to leave the state to seek opportunity elsewhere (Lefler 434). After 1835 settlement began to expand rapidly in the western piedmont zones, and an increasing sectionalism developed as political power also began to shift westward. The new centralization of power led to reforms in the tax system and the spread of state services to rural areas. This period of progress, however, came to an abrupt halt with the outbreak of the Civil War—a conflict that destroyed much of the state's wealth and took the lives of 40,000 of its inhabitants (Lefler 436). Once the war ended, moreover, the state had to adjust to the emancipation of an estimated 350,000 slaves in its efforts not only to rebuild the economy but to provide services and political rights to all inhabitants.

After the end of Reconstruction, the Democrats won control of the legislature and political influence shifted completely from the agricultural establishment of the eastern region to the industrial and business interests of the west. During the period prior to the Great Depression, thousands of miles of railroads were built in the state and the expansion of manufacturing and textiles grew rapidly. The economy of the east lagged behind that in the west, causing the majority of the region's small farmers to suffer economically. Moreover, the Democratic establishment repealed suffrage for blacks in 1900, causing the large population of African-Americans concentrated in the east to suffer disproportionately from the region's decline.

In the boom period after the end of World War II, the legislature moved to expand economic development and the delivery of services to disadvantaged areas of the state. There were intensified efforts to diversify industry and improve agricultural efficiency and productivity. These efforts resulted, however, in a drastic decline in the number of farms in the eastern region, forcing an increasing number of landless laborers to seek work in textile and small manufacturing plants in other parts of the state (Lefler 436). The 1970s and 1980s have seen an expansion in the east of poultry and hog processing plants attracted by the availability of a large pool of inexpensive labor. Today this industry is one of the major employers of nonfarm labor in the eastern regions of North Carolina and Virginia (Freedman).

Historically, the eastern regions of North Carolina and Virginia have been poor, and that situation remains unchanged today. While they were among the first areas settled, and while some large landholders in the colonial period accumulated vast fortunes and exercised considerable political influence, the region since then has been and continues to be dominated by small farmers and poor, landless laborers. Today most of the eastern region of both states is officially designated as rural, although there is considerable diversity in that designation.

Three predominant population patterns prevail. The coastal rural counties of the region are inhabited largely by whites of English descent who have, until recently, been isolated from the mainland. Residents of these counties are involved in marine extractive activities, shipbuilding, seasonal agriculture, and, increasingly, tourist-related occupations. In addition, these counties are presently experiencing a boom in development spurred by the construction of recreational and retirement housing.

The inland rural counties, formerly characterized by a plantation agriculture system focused on cotton and tobacco, are largely inhabited today by small farmers and landless laborers. As agriculture has declined in profitability, many white landowners have emigrated, leaving behind a largely black and impoverished population in these counties. Some of these laborers were able to find employment in textile and manufacturing plants, but as these industries have become less competitive on a global scale, plant closings have led to a second wave of large-scale unemployment in the region. Finally, there is a small number of inland, urban-nucleus counties in this region. These counties have a central city, usually with a population of 50,000 or less, surrounded by rural zones of agricultural activity. Many impoverished inhabitants of the rural counties are moving into the urban areas to seek employment opportunities which, more often than not, are unavailable to them.

About 25 percent of the population of this eastern region lives below the poverty line, compared to 14.4 percent nationally (Freedman 41). Median annual family income in the inland rural counties is $13,502 as compared to $19,917 nationally (Freedman 41). Perhaps a more striking illustration of the level of poverty in the region is shown by a comparison of county figures within North Carolina. In 1980 the average per capita annual income in the state was $7,832, which was 82 percent of the national average. Of the thirty-two counties in the eastern region of North Carolina, thirty fell below the state average, and ten of the inland rural and predominantly black counties had average per capita annual incomes of less than $6,000 (Wilms and Powell 8). For Indians in the region the figures are even worse, with an estimated 44 percent of the Lumbee population, for example, reporting a per capita annual income below the poverty level (Red Corn).

This extreme poverty, combined with the relative isolation, low educational levels of the population, and the lack of infrastructure to attract new industry, has led to a massive emigration of younger and more able-bodied people. Consequently, the percentage of the population which is elderly, disabled, or living in large families is rising (Friedman 42). Many of these residents are poor and unable to work, and the proportion of those dependent on some form of public assistance has grown. Further complicating the situation is that the entire eastern region of North Carolina, as well as that of southeastern Virginia, is an officially designated "health manpower shortage area." Although the average physician to patient ratio in the state of North Carolina improved from 1 per 911 people in 1978 to 1 per 637 people in 1987, the ratio in the eastern counties declined dramatically. There were more than 1,000 practicing physicians in the eastern 32 counties of North Carolina in 1980; however, the distribution of these physicians in the population varied dramatically from a ratio of 1 for every 539 people in the urban-nucleus counties, to an average of 1 for every 3,550 in many inland black counties, to a low of 1 for 9,486 and 16,117 and none at all for 25,000 in the three most isolated counties (Wilms and Powell 17; *What If . . . ?* A4; *Statistics on Physician Availability*).

In addition to the lack of care, the health profile of the region is a poor one. In 1988 the region had one of the highest infant mortality rates (12.6 per 1,000 live births) in the nation; and, even more disturbing, nonwhites averaged 18.7 deaths per 1,000 live births, a rate far worse than that found in all of the industrialized nations of the West and in many Third World countries (Bloch A1; *North Carolina Vital Statistics* 2–1). In addition, the incidence of hypertension, obesity, diabetes mellitus, arteriosclerosis, cancer, chronic obstructive pulmonary disease, tuberculosis, renal calculi, and cardiovascular disease far exceeds the national average (Fabsitz and Feinleib). This is consistent with the greater incidence and prevalence of chronic illness in rural areas in general (Norton and McManus).

Clearly, then, the long history of geographic isolation in largely rural areas, coupled with the lack of access to educational opportunities and government services occasioned by extreme poverty, has forced the inhabitants of the eastern region to be self-reliant in meeting their needs. Because cultural traditions have survived relatively intact in this area and because many inhabitants have had to rely on their own knowledge and skills in treating illness, it is not surprising that traditional medicine continues to flourish in this population. Although efforts have been made to extend biomedical services in the area, many inhabitants of the eastern counties do not have access to them. Moreover, those who do often continue to rely on traditional techniques, sometimes using them in conjunction with biomedical ones.

In a recent study Mitchell and Mathews interviewed 900 older adults sampled randomly in proportion to the distribution of racial and ethnic groups and of the sexes in the general population of twelve counties in eastern North Carolina. Part of the survey was designed to elicit information about the prevalence of traditional medical beliefs in the population and about the extent to which traditional practitioners and remedies were utilized and for what purposes. Preliminary results show that, on average across the twelve counties, 35 percent of the population surveyed is actively using some form of traditional or alternative medicine, most often in conjunction with some form of biomedicine. The traditional practitioners consulted include more exotic ones such as root doctors (specialists who can cause and cure illness with the use of magic spells known as "roots"), herbalists and palmists, together with more generally familiar and "orthodox" ones such as religious faith healers, ministers, chiropractors, pharmacists, health food vendors, and less formally, influential community members, particularly funeral home directors. Nonmedical remedies used include various foods and beverages, herbal potions, prayer, protective amulets, and magical spells or "roots." Medical resources used in nonmedically prescribed ways include a host of over-the-counter medications and more old-fashioned tonics or patent medicines employed locally both to cure and prevent illness (Mitchell and Mathews 1, 2). As anticipated, the rates of traditional use varied across the different types of counties. They were lowest, comprising 10–15 percent of the population surveyed, in the two urban-nucleus counties; average, comprising 35 percent of the population surveyed, in the coastal white counties; and highest, comprising 50–60 percent of the population surveyed, in the inland, predominantly black counties.

Mitchell and Mathews are among the first to document statistically the continued use of traditional medical practices in a randomly surveyed population (see also Roebuck and Quan). The investigators initially expected, in line with current assumptions about the general decline of traditional beliefs during increasing modernization and urbanization, that such use patterns would be found in only 10 percent of the population. Obviously, however, traditional medical beliefs and practices are still important to the region's inhabitants, and this surprising persistence raises the question of why they continue to exist, even when biomedical alternatives are available.

In chapter one in this volume, David Hufford responds to this question by discussing some of the reasons for the continued influence of traditional medicine in various parts of the world today. He suggests that such beliefs and practices represent "a universal set of efforts to cope with illness in ways that go beyond—but do not necessarily conflict with—what modern medicine has to offer" (15). He argues, consequently, that folk medical beliefs and practices are of major importance to scientific medicine because they are a crucial part of the foundation from which patients derive their attitudes and decisions with respect to biomedical care. A brief examination of the ways in which traditional medicines generally differ in philosophy and practice from biomedicine can help suggest avenues for the development of methods and procedures that accomplish the goal Hufford specifies of finding a "reasonable way of taking folk medicine into account in the clinic" (14).

As Bannerman et al. point out, all medical practice was what we now call traditional until the beginning of the nineteenth century, when the "great philosophical upheaval of the renaissance began to introduce Cartesian scientific materialism into all human activities and noticeably into the theory and practice of medicine" (11). The development of scientific medicine involved a shift from the mind-body holism of traditional systems to a dualistic conception that is posited to be the outgrowth of the following: first, a scientific method which tends to break complex phenomena into their component parts and deal with each in isolation (Bannerman et al. 11); second, the pharmacologic goal of isolating the active principles of disease coupled with the physician's desire to find efficient treatments for the physical causes of disease (Bannerman et al. 11); and, finally, the necessity of communication in a scientific medical language (Hall and Bourne 141). Over time, physicians became less involved in handling the complex life situations that patients often perceived as relevant to the diagnosis and treatment of physical illness. Consequently, while scientific medicine met with remarkable success in treating disorders caused by infectious agents, by poor sanitation and nutrition, and by personal injury, it has been markedly less successful in handling the effects of chronic, degenerative conditions and in resolving psychiatric and psychosomatic complaints where behavioral, emotional, and spiritual factors play a major role in etiology and outcome (Bannerman et al. 11; Hall and Bourne 141; Wintrob).

In contrast, traditional systems are based on a mind-body holism that is usually embedded in a society's view of personhood and the relationship of the individual to natural and supernatural realms. In such systems, the divisions between medicine and other cultural institutions such as religion, politics, social organization, and economics are not well demarcated. Foster and Anderson, therefore, argue that the efficacy of such systems must be evaluated in terms of their "ability to successfully play roles that lie far beyond the cure of illness and the maintenance of health" (125).

In such systems, for example, the alleviation of physical symptoms may be of secondary importance to the goal of restoring the individual to social and/or spiritual harmony with the group. This goal is reflected in the frequent preoccupation of individual patients with finding out, as Wintrob writes, "*why* rather than *how* a particular person fell ill, progressed toward recovery, or died" (318). Such a preoccupation is, in turn, rooted in explanations for illness that are seemingly irrational and illogical, emphasizing as they do a combination of magical, supernatural, and social causes for illness. Yet as Foster and Anderson point out, the curing ceremonies and treatments congruent with these expectations often function to provide people with explanations for unexplainable phenomena, to exert a measure of control in restraining deviant behaviors that violate social norms, to reintegrate a deviant or mentally ill person into the community, to provide a therapeutic public confession that engenders emotional catharsis and a sharing of guilt for the patient, and to give psychosocial support to those in need (126–28). Moreover, empirically derived herbal pharmacopoeias may be effective in relieving distress for a number of routine illnesses, although comparative studies which attempt to document the efficacy along with the dangers of such remedies are few (Croom's essay, chapter eight, is an important addition to this literature).

The fact that a serious reawakening of interest in the emotional, spiritual, and irrational aspects of health is occurring today in precisely those societies that have a long experience with scientific medicine indicates that many of the psychosocial needs addressed in traditional systems remain unmet in the biomedical sphere (Bannerman et al. 12; McGuire). This is not to claim, as Hufford points out, that traditional medical systems are somehow better or more effective than biomedicine or that biomedical practitioners should try to be all things to all patients. Rather, the authors in this volume view the serious study of the contributions of traditional medicine to modern practice as a way of providing lessons for a more humane and culturally sensitive healing.

In chapter two Richard Blaustein presents a précis of the articles to follow and delineates the contributions of the various disciplines represented to a collaborative model of inquiry. As a folklorist with an academic appointment in family medicine and psychiatry, Blaustein is doubly aware of the difficulties inherent in attempting to grasp the pluralistic approach most Americans have to health care. He argues for the importance of a multidisciplinary perspective if we are "to realize once again the fundamental interdependence of mind and body, individual and society, humanity and the natural world" (40). Each discipline approaches the study of human behavior from a unique theoretical perspective, employs different types of research methods, generates different kinds of data, and, as a result, provides different solutions to common problems.

For example, folklorists who document traditional beliefs and practices tend to focus analysis on the interactions between respondents. Consequently, they do not usually quantify responses to standardized questionnaires as is common in some social science and clinical research. Yet their data are no less valuable as a result and may, in the end, be more useful than survey research in suggesting ways to bridge the cultural and communication gap between physicians and patients. Similarly, anthropologists tend to rely on qualitative methods to determine how traditional beliefs and practices derive from an integrated cultural and social system and function to meet the needs of that system's members. Their data are useful in demonstrating how such beliefs structure the expectations and behaviors exhibited by patients in the clinical setting and in suggesting ways that such beliefs can be integrated into biomedical practice. Clinicians and scientists, on the other hand, use a range of experimental methods including epidemiologic research, natural experiments, clinical trials, and case-control studies to measure the efficacy of their own practices by delineating, in part, the impact of traditional beliefs and practices on the overall effectiveness of biomedical techniques. In other instances, clinical practitioners use carefully documented case studies to explore the effect on treatment outcomes of a patient's medical and family history, attitudes toward illness, interactions with medical staff, and compliance with care. Such case studies, as Peter Lichstein shows in chapter six, provide insights that enable clinicians to formulate strategies for promoting more effective therapeutic alliances with patients from different sociocultural backgrounds. Ultimately, the integrated picture that emerges from a multidisciplinary approach will provide a template for planners who have as their goal the development of community-based interventions for health promotion and disease prevention.

This multidisciplinary volume is intended to serve a varied audience including folklorists, anthropologists, health scientists, physicians, and other health care specialists in several ways. It provides illuminating commentaries on the major forms of naturopathic and magico-religious medicine currently practiced in the United States and on the physical, social, and cultural contexts in the focus region. It documents and explains the persistence of these traditions in our modern technological society. It examines the bases of folk medical concepts of illness and treatment and the efficacy of particular cures. It provides extensive bibliographical documentation of the scope and variety of research on traditional medicine. And, perhaps most significantly, it suggests a model for collaborative research that can be replicated wherever scholars in different disciplines are united by a common interest in this important dimension of human culture and are committed to the serious, open-minded exploration of attitudes and behaviors that have often been dismissed as mere ignorance or quackery.

References

Bannerman, Robert H., John Burton, and Ch'en Wen-Chieh. Introduction. *Traditional Medicine and Health Care Coverage.* Ed. Robert Bannerman, John Burton, and Ch'en Wen-Chieh. Geneva: World Health Organization (WHO), 1983. 9–13.

Bloch, Judy. "Edgecombe is Battling to Save Its Babies." *News and Observer* (Raleigh, N.C.). April 1, 1990: A1, A12.

Fabsitz, R., and M. Feinleib. "Geographic Patterns in County Mortality Rates from Cardiovascular Diseases." *American Journal of Epidemiology* 111.3 (1980): 315–28.

Foster, George M., and Barbara G. Anderson. *Medical Anthropology.* New York: John Wiley and Sons, 1978.

Freedman, Deborah. "An Isolated Pocket of Poverty in Northeastern North Carolina." *How the Poor Would Remedy Poverty.* Washington, D.C.: Coalition on Human Needs, 1986. 41–51.

Hall, Arthur L., and Peter G. Bourne. "Indigenous Therapists in a Southern Black Urban Community." *Archives of General Psychiatry* 28 (1973): 137–42.

Hughes, Charles C. "Medical Care: Ethnomedicine." *Health and the Human Condition: Perspectives on Medical Anthropology.* Ed. Michael H. Logan and Edward E. Hunt, Jr. Belmont, Calif.: Wadsworth, 1978. 150–57.

Lefler, Hugh T. "North Carolina." *The Encyclopedia Americana International Edition.* 1990 ed.

Lefler, Hugh T., and William S. Powell. *Colonial North Carolina.* New York: Charles Scribner's Sons, 1973.

McGuire, Meredith B., with the assistance of Debra Kantor. *Ritual Healing in Suburban America.* New Brunswick: Rutgers University Press, 1988.

Mahler, Halfdan. Foreword. *Traditional Medicine and Health Care Coverage.* Ed. Robert Bannerman, John Burton, and Ch'en Wen-Chieh. Geneva: WHO, 1983. 7–9.

Merrens, Harry Roy. *Colonial North Carolina in the Eighteenth Century.* Chapel Hill: University of North Carolina Press, 1964.

Mitchell, James P., and Holly F. Mathews. "Alternative Health Care Use among the Rural Elderly in Eastern North Carolina." Unpublished report, 1991.

North Carolina State. Department of Environment, Health, and Natural Resources. *North Carolina Vital Statistics.* Vol. 1. Raleigh, N.C.: Division of Statistics and Information Services, 1988.

Norton, C. H., and M. A. McManus. "Background Tables on Demographic Characteristics, Health Status, and Health Services Utilization." *Health Services Research* 23.6 (1989): 725–50.

Red Corn, J. *American Indians of the South Atlantic Region by County.* American Indian Census and Statistical Data Project. Publication no. 82-102070. Springfield, Va.: National Technological Information Service, 1980.

Rights, Douglas L. *The American Indian in North Carolina.* Winston-Salem, N.C.: Douglas F. Blair, 1957.

Roebuck, Julian, and Robert Quan. "Health-Care Practices in the American Deep South." *Marginal Medicine.* Ed. Roy Wallis and Peter Morley. New York: Free, 1976. 141–61.

Statistics on Physician Availability in Eastern North Carolina. Greenville, N.C.: Center for Health Services Research and Development, East Carolina University School of Medicine, 1988.

United States Department of Commerce. Bureau of the Census. *North Carolina Final Population and Housing Unit Counts.* Census of Population and Housing Advance Reports. PHC 80-V-35. Washington, D.C.: GPO, 1982.

Wetmore, Ruth Y. *First on the Land: The North Carolina Indians.* Winston-Salem, N.C.: John F. Blair, 1975.

"What If . . . ? School of Medicine has Contributed." *Daily Reflector* (Greenville, N.C.). April 3, 1990: A4.

Wilms, Douglas C., and William G. Powell. *Eastern North Carolina: An Atlas of Demographic and Economic Trends.* Greenville, N.C.: Regional Development Institute of East Carolina University, 1983.

Wintrob, Ronald M. "The Influence of Others: Witchcraft and Rootwork as Explanations of Behavior Disturbances." *The Journal of Nervous and Mental Disease* 156.5 (1973): 318–26.

1. Folk Medicine in Contemporary America

David J. Hufford

It is my purpose in this essay to situate the regional folk medicine studies in this book within the medical and the national contexts.

Folk medicine is defined by contrast to modern, scientific medicine, the "official" medicine of the modern world. We say that a belief or practice is folk medicine because we recognize that it is not official. This enormous and diverse body of unofficial health culture is the foundation from which many patients derive their attitudes and decisions about medical care. However, this fact is not obvious from the medical perspective, and even when it has been recognized, the development of a reasonable way of taking folk medicine into account in the clinic is a complex job. I have been a member of the Behavioral Science Department of the Pennsylvania State University College of Medicine since 1974, and my suggestions here come from that experience of medical teaching, research, and consultation.

The national context is equally important. The stereotype of folk medicine associates it with populations isolated from the modern cultural mainstream. This is partly because of the erroneous assumption that modern medicine inevitably replaces all other cultural health resources as soon as it is available. Therefore, the documentation of folk medical traditions within any particular region, especially one that is rural, is often perceived as setting that region apart from the national culture. This notion of folk medicine as marginal is as unfortunate as it is incorrect (Hufford 242–53). The traditions documented in this book are cultural elements that North Carolina and Virginia patients *have in common* with patients elsewhere. As I shall discuss below, folk medicine is not restricted to any single region or demographically defined group. Instead, it represents a universal set of efforts to cope with illness in ways that go beyond—but do not necessarily conflict with—what modern medicine has to offer.

This is a central part of my argument for the medical importance of folk medicine. We are not dealing here with a few surviving vestiges of premodern medical thought. We are dealing with vigorous community resources for coping with illness that show no sign of being in decline. Both folklorists and health professionals *need* to recognize and strive to understand this fact if their analyses are to be sound and if their practice is to be effective.

The Extent and Relationship of American Healing Systems

The following five points are essential to a discussion of healing systems. Although they may seem obvious at first glance, they are nonetheless frequently overlooked when feelings begin to run high on matters of health.

American Healing Systems are Numerous and Varied

In the United States today there exist a great variety of traditions of healing. Some of these have the relief of physical disease as their primary goal; examples of such systems are modern conventional medicine and homeopathy. Others focus primarily on the prevention of disease, for example, conservative chiropractic; and others on the enhancement of health, for example, health foods and organic farming. Still others have a completely different primary goal: most religious healing practices exist within traditions in which salvation is the primary goal, while the healing of physical and mental disease is prominent but clearly of secondary importance.

Some of these systems occupy firmly established "official" positions in our society, such as conventional medicine and osteopathy. Others are definitely unofficial or "folk" in their status, as is the case with Pennsylvania German powwowing or the North Carolina burn-healing tradition discussed by Kirkland and Sammons in chapters three and four. Some are necessarily in conflict because they are based on diametrically opposed sets of assumptions, as Christian Science and medical science. Others, such as the tradition of prayer for healing in most Christian denominations and most forms of physical treatment of disease, are so accustomed to one another that neither clergy nor health care personnel normally think of themselves as in competition.

Some of these systems appear relatively new, but most of them are historically related to older traditions, as chiropractic is related to traditions of "bonesetting," much of the modern health food movement is related to ancient folk herbalism, and conventional medicine is the culmination of many strands of official and folk healing traditions spanning centuries. The current tension among these systems, especially between modern, conventional medicine and most other healing traditions, is sometimes characterized as a distinctly modern situation, but it too is a continuation of past struggles and requires an historical perspective to be properly understood.

This book discusses several important, representative systems found in North Carolina and Virginia, but these do not exhaust the possible examples. The fact is that we live in a pluralistic health culture, although one particular form of healing tradition has become the primary official one over the past eighty years or so. The variety of healing traditions shows no sign of decreasing, and a major purpose of this book is to seek an understanding of the regional sources and nature of this diversity and to look for ways in which such an understanding can work to the advantage of both practitioners of healing and their clients.

"Rational" and "Logical" Do Not Equal "Correct" or "True"

When discussing health systems with any group, I always begin by noting that most of them (from conventional medicine to psychic healing to herbalism to faith healing) are rational systems of thought. Immediately, I encounter an argument to the effect that this cannot be because such and such a system is *not correct.* Perhaps this judgment of correctness is right and perhaps not. But that judgment is not relevant to this point. "Rational" simply means based on the coherent use of human reason. Reasoning, including formal deductive logic, cannot guarantee truth. If assumptions, criteria for the admission of evidence and observations, differ, then the same kind of reasoning may lead to very different conclusions.

The importance of recognizing the rationality of a system of ideas is that it gives people with different viewpoints a common ground for discussion. A surgeon and a faith healer can rather easily be brought to understand the logic of each other's thought if each will listen to a straightforward description of the assumptions and observations involved. This understanding can lead to a reasonable discussion that can work to the advantage of each and, even more important, to the advantage of a patient who may be seeking help from both simultaneously. Because emotions tend to be so strong in such discussions, it may be necessary for a third party to help communicate the straightforward description—for example, a medical folklorist or anthropologist (or the patient in the middle)—but it is still not that complicated a task to accomplish.

"Understanding" Does not Equal "Agreement"

When contemplating a request to *understand* someone else's very different point of view, there is a certain amount of uneasiness, arising from the possibility that this understanding might mean agreement. Certainly when agreement between opposing points of view is possible, it is most likely to be gained by understanding. However, it is perfectly possible (and rational) that two parties may come to a fairly complete understanding of each other's viewpoints and still neither be able to agree nor to disprove the other's point. If that is so, what good is this understanding? Together with the grasping of the other's logic, this understanding makes possible reasonable discussion and negotiation. As I shall argue below, the removal of conflict between very different healing systems is possible to a certain extent in some cases. However, just as important is the ability to recognize those differences that are irreconcilable and find the basis for a rational negotiation that will reduce the negative effects of the conflict on individual patients and the public in general.

Honesty. Sometimes in discussions of the need to understand and respect the beliefs of patients, and at times to accommodate them in treatment, health professionals develop the impression that they are being asked to pretend. This is not the case. It would be neither ethical nor practical to pretend agreement with beliefs that one does not share. But agreement is not the primary thing most patients seek on this subject. They wish to have those beliefs that they see as relevant to their health and treatment listened to, responded to honestly, and taken into account in planning treatment. Such attitudes are prevalent among the individuals whose case histories on North Carolina rootworking traditions Mathews and Lichstein discuss in chapters five and six. And another excellent example can be seen when a Jehovah's Witness tells his surgeon he will not accept blood transfusions. He doesn't expect to convince the surgeon that transfusions are bad. He expects the surgeon to understand his religious basis for rejecting transfusions, to explain how this will affect his case, and then to honestly abide by his clearly stated wishes. These wishes may be taken directly from the entire teaching of the Witnesses, or they may be some personal variation of those teachings. Whatever they are, though, the Witness has a right to have his belief and wishes heard (the surgeon can never assume that he or she knows in advance exactly what an individual Witness's specific position will be), to be understood, and to be acted on.

It may seem at first glance that such an example, rooted as it is in the patient's formal religious commitment, is a special kind of exception. However, beliefs not officially derived from a religious institution—but part of the patient's lived world view—are often as firmly held, as personally important, and as ethically salient as those that are.

Alternative Health Systems Are Extremely Vigorous and Persistent

From the point of view of conventional medicine, the need for understanding and negotiation with alternative views of health has not seemed very urgent in this century. It has been assumed that alternatives were in the process of dying out in the face of modern medical technology. By the beginning of the 1980s, however, it is clear that this prediction is off the mark. Interest in and use of alternatives to modern medicine (often in addition to medical care rather than as pure alternatives) have, if anything, increased.

In 1988 I had the opportunity to document this startling fact with regard to cancer, while participating in a project of the U.S. Congress, Office of Technology Assessment, intended to lead to the objective evaluation of unorthodox cancer treatments. My research involved both literature review and fieldwork, but here I shall only comment on what the literature showed concerning hard evidence on the prevalence of folk medicine. The best quantitative study published to date was carried out by Barrie Cassileth and her colleagues at the University of Pennsylvania. This study involved 304 patients at the University of Pennsylvania Cancer Center in Philadelphia and 356 patients of unorthodox practitioners in the Philadelphia area. Among the Cancer Center patients, 13 percent were currently using or had used some form of folk medical treatment. Among the entire group of 660 patients, contrary to conventional expectations, "Patients on unorthodox treatment . . . tended to be white ($p<0.00001$) and better educated ($p<0.00001$) than patients on conventional treatment only" (Cassileth et al. 107). The treatments used ranged from herbs to dietary changes to healing prayer and unorthodox medicine such as "immune therapies." The design of this study, like most other quantitative work, used a conservative definition that did not elicit many reports of self-treatment. Since self-treatment is very common in folk medicine, we must assume that these quantitative assessments yield very conservative figures. A colleague, Peter Houts, and I recently carried out a survey of folk medicine used by 628 cancer patients in central Pennsylvania, using a design intended to include self-treatments, so long as they were undertaken to actually combat the patient's cancer. We found that this approach yielded a utilization rate of more than 70 percent. The most frequently used methods were spiritual and religious, a kind of tactic that is almost universal in folk medical traditions. For example, 73 percent used some form of prayer and 7 percent attended some kind of formal healing service. Other kinds of methods used included visual imagery techniques (17 percent) and dietary strategies (11.3 percent), both of which are prominent elements in a variety of folk medical traditions (unpublished data).

Several other quantitative studies have been carried out on this topic within the past twelve years. All have found significant utilization of folk medical treatments among cancer patients ranging from a low of 6 percent reported among pediatric patients (Copeland) to substantially higher incidence than that reported by Cassileth et al. For example, the 23 percent reported by Newell et al. in 1986. Of those that have reported characteristics associated with utilization, all have supported the findings of Cassileth et al. For example, Newell et al. found that "the user of unorthodox cancer treatments was likely to be younger, better educated, more knowledgeable concerning cancer treatments," and Mooney found that "Users were more action-oriented, consulted more information sources, and were more familiar with treatment options." Studies outside the United States suggest that utilization of unorthodox treatments is even more common in other countries (Arkko et al.; Dady et al.; Pruyn). Such studies find a variety of practices ranging from the older, often ethnically linked traditions such as *curanderismo* in the Southwest to modern, "New Age," holistic approaches. These different traditions tend, as one would expect, to be utilized by different patient groups. However, the modern-looking approaches have strong, often explicit, connections with the older forms (as holistic health advocates seek to incorporate shamanism, herbalism, and other ancient techniques within a modern context), so this distinction should not be exaggerated.

Some might assume that these findings of high prevalence, especially among mainstream patients, is peculiar to cancer treatment. However, all indications, both quantitative and ethnographic, are that reliance on folk medicine is similar for all health matters. For example, in the spring of 1986 a study carried out under contract with the Department of Health and Human Services conducted a national survey of the attitudes that the "non-institutionalized, adult population" of the United States held toward the utilization of "questionable" treatments for disease in general and for arthritis and cancer in particular (Lou Harris and Associates). The general questions were asked of a national cross-sectional sample of 1,514, and the final cancer patient sample included 297 persons. The authors note that the questions focused on a "restricted domain of fifteen treatment areas, in which products have been systematically classified as scientifically acceptable or questionable" and therefore "these estimates should be treated as conservative" (ii). Certainly folk medical practices were counted as questionable in this study, but no doubt a great many were not asked about. The authors report that the general population is *much more* likely than cancer patients to use questionable treatments (26.6 percent), 21 percent having used them within the past year as compared to about 15 percent of cancer patients who are using such treatments. "College graduates seem more likely than those without a degree to use treatments that are questionable" (v), but the authors note that in other ways those who use questionable treatments are demographically indistinguishable from the general population.

Although research on folk medicine has been ethnographic much more often than quantitative, it is clear that what quantitative work has been done strongly supports the conclusion of folklorists and anthropologists that folk medicine is vigorous, persistent, and prevalent in the United States. This survey research also supports the observation that folk medicine is not linked to a particular segment of the population or that it survives only among the "ignorant."

In some specific cases, medicine may need to continue efforts to reduce the influence of these alternatives, or to alter the nature of their practice. That is, there are some for which a good case may be made that they are actually harmful. Nonetheless, it must be granted that in almost one century of intense efforts, bolstered by substantial legal and financial assistance, conventional medicine has not even begun to wipe out nonofficial healing practices and beliefs. This observation will be granted both by those who support and those who oppose these efforts at eradication. Therefore, the need to understand and to be able to negotiate concerning the issues involved seems very pressing. As early as the mid-1970s, articles in medical journals had begun to grant this point with regard to one of the systems with which it has been most at odds, chiropractic. An article in the *New England Journal of Medicine* by Gregory J. Firman, M.D., J.D., and Michael S. Goldstein, Ph.D., "The Future of Chiropractic" (639–42), concluded that "the role of chiropractic within the health-care system will remain stable in the future" (639). Or, as an article in *Medical Economics* by A. J. Vogel put it, "It's Time to Take Chiropractors Seriously" (76–85). This is true not only of the most highly visible instances, such as chiropractic. It is, in fact, time to take folk medicine in general seriously.

Modern Technological Medicine Is Extremely Vigorous and Persistent

It is certainly true that modern medicine has come under a great deal of criticism, perhaps more in recent years than earlier in this century. However, medicine has demonstrated remarkable effectiveness in treating certain kinds of diseases and has effectively captured the central position as North America's official form of health care. This does not mean, however, that visits to medical doctors constitute the most numerous health-related acts in our society, although we sometimes speak as though this were the case. The best estimates of the involvement of official medical contacts in health complaints place these contacts at 10 percent or fewer of the health actions taken by people who are self-defined as sick.[1] The other 90 percent of health actions include the explicit use of other healing traditions, but are not limited to them. They also include the taking of patent medicines such as aspirin, decisions to try bed rest, and so on. However, even when the actions are purely self-care in nature, they often involve decisions that are based on information derived from alternative systems (whether folk wisdom such as "feed a cold, starve a fever," or more recent ideas such as taking vitamin C tablets for a cold).

Nonetheless, when symptoms persist or are severe, or when a serious injury occurs, a visit to the medical doctor is the most common action for most Americans. Even for those who have another first line resource—for example, a visit to a powwow or to a chiropractor, or to community healers such as those discussed in the following essays—a medical visit is a very common second or third resort. This fact, coupled with medicine's close working relationship with our society's governmental systems (such as state departments of health, and the federal Food and Drug Administration) seems to indicate clearly that modern medicine is here to stay in a recognizable form and at the official center of our society's health care establishment.

I make this observation because there are some critics of medicine who have predicted a withering of conventional medicine in the face of popular alternatives in a way reminiscent of medicine's prediction that *its* competition would soon die out. There is no doubt that cultural change, including changes in our health institutions, will continue in modern society. However, the likelihood that a "new age medicine" will achieve ascendancy and replace conventional medicine in the foreseeable future seems very remote. To paraphrase the above quote about chiropractic, alternative healing systems must also take modern medicine seriously.

It seems that a state of dynamic tension in an essentially pluralistic health culture will continue for a long time. This book is in large part devoted to understanding the implications of that pluralism and finding ways of promoting rational discourse among the systems and individuals who make up this pluralistic mosaic. From this perspective conventional medicine, like those folk medicine traditions discussed here, is an "alternative healing system," "alternative" being a thoroughly relative form.

Healing Systems

"The health care system" conjures up a picture of the scientific, clinical, bureaucratic, and governmental institution that is modern medicine. The conventional picture of folk and other nonmedical healing traditions consists of loosely associated batches of belief and practice, not systems at all. However, this is part of what is wrong with our view of the varied healing traditions that coexist with modern medicine, and most of which substantially predate it. There certainly are outdated bits of medical thought still in circulation, and there are a variety of mistaken ideas about health just as there are about any subject. However, it is a grave error to assume that nonmedical healing traditions are composed primarily of such mistaken and outdated notions. It was this idea of survivalism that gave rise to the conventional expectation, early in this century, that as science in general and medical science in particular progressed—in technical knowledge, in availability, and in dissemination through education—alternative beliefs and practices would die out. The technological progress, increased availability, and educational dissemination have all been breathtaking during this century, and yet modern medicine appears to be under more competition from a variety of alternatives today than it was one hundred years ago.

In understanding this intriguing historical fact, and in understanding the various healing traditions themselves, the first need is to recognize these traditions as *systems.* A system is a collection of parts among which there are meaningful relationships. This is true of the parts that make up such healing traditions as rootwork, naturopathy, *Santería,* and all of the others that persist in living form.

Two of the most important characteristics of systems are their complexity (that is, the number of parts they contain) and their integration (the number of orderly relationships among those parts); for example, a jigsaw puzzle heaped on a table may be seen as a system—it remains at one level of complexity but becomes more integrated as the pieces are put together. Although most alternative healing systems may be less complex than modern medicine, considering the scientific information explosion, many of them are at least as integrated. This is important because integration tends to increase stability. Perhaps even more important is the fact that one can only understand the logic of a cultural system by recognizing and understanding the connections among its parts. It is impossible, for example, to understand the naturopathic preference for naturally derived vitamins over their pure synthetic counterparts, or for herbal treatments instead of isolated or synthetic doses of the pharmacologically active component of the herb (for example, foxglove leaf instead of digoxin), by examining it purely from the perspective of the modern medical system. Seen this way the preference seems to have no meaningful connection to anything else and therefore appears arbitrary. However, when this preference is viewed from within the naturopathic system a great many orderly connections may be seen between it and a large number of naturopathic understandings about the world and humanity's place in it. The single idea can suddenly be seen as part of coherent, mutually supportive observations and ideas rather than an isolated "error." Seeing the preference in this way may not lead a person grounded in medical science to agree with the preference, but it may result in increased understanding and rational discussion.

Cultural Health Systems and Individual Health Systems

There are two ways of looking at any system of ideas embedded in culture: the ideal overview, and the embodiment of such ideal conceptualizations within the lives and thoughts of individuals. Neither is more correct than the other, both being necessary to a balanced view of the operation of culture and its expression in particular lives. Whenever we make such statements as "modern medicine demonstrates that . . .," "homeopathy is based on . . .," or "rootworkers believe that . . .," we are speaking of idealized cultural systems. These idealized descriptions are based on the collation of many individual views. To the extent that the views of the majority, or at least the most influential, of the adherents of a point of view have been summed up in these statements, they are useful. But they always remain an intellectual device. A system of ideas cannot act; a tradition cannot *believe* something. It is individuals who act, believe, and express the views we conflate to create our descriptions of these traditions. When we take the time (and it *does* take a great deal of time) to find out just what an individual believes and what he or she does, it is often possible to say this individual is an adherent of a particular cultural system. However, no individual ever *completely* replicates a single tradition. There are always idiosyncrasies and there are usually signs of influence from other traditions. The most conventional and orthodox of cultural systems always include some diversity of opinion and always show some sign of influence from outside themselves, at least in our heterogeneous cultural milieux.

When we identify an individual as an "herbalist," or as a "Charismatic Christian," we are justified in immediately forming some hypotheses about how that person is likely to feel and act on certain health issues. However, if we do not immediately begin a discussion with the individual to find out where his or her views coincide with our idealized view of that system we are guilty of stereotypical thinking. Clinically we must know that not all Jehovah's Witnesses refuse all blood products; not all (or even most) Charismatics believe they must "claim a healing" and refuse medical treatment while "standing on the word of God"; not all users of Laetrile refuse chemotherapy; not all (or even most) clients of chiropractors refuse medical treatment for acute conditions; and some Christian Scientists will submit to surgery. And the older forms of folk medicine are even less commonly found in direct conflict with modern medicine.

Our understanding of cultural health systems must be somewhat like our understanding of other groups. Men are much more likely than women to have heart attacks, but some women do have heart attacks and some men in their fifties with chest pain are suffering from hiatal hernia or musculoskeletal problems. An avowed vegetarian may be developing a vitamin B-12 deficiency or consuming exactly the nutrients that every medical doctor *and* every naturopath wish their clients would consume.

Scholars of health systems, practitioners of healing, and patients themselves must keep this distinction in mind or they will eventually fall prey to the same grave errors to which all stereotypical thinking leads. From the patients' point of view the fact that a healer is identified as an "M.D." or as a "rootworker" or as a "spirit filled healer" must be only a useful beginning in determining whether this is the person to whom they wish to entrust an important part of their health care. Both practitioners and clients, if they wish to be rational in their selection of their health resources, must move quickly from hypothetical knowledge about a person, based on a labeled connection with a health system or school of thought, to specific knowledge of what this label means in the case of the person with whom they are dealing.

Do They Work?

The first question people want to ask when the subject of healing practices comes up, especially alternative healing practices, concerns efficacy. Which things work and which things don't? These are natural questions, but they are considerably more difficult to answer than is generally realized. There are two ways to set about answering them in a systematic way. The first is the one that has been done most often by scholars, and it consists of comparing an alternative practice to the practices current in medicine. We could call this the theoretical approach. If an alternative practice is recognizably very similar to a medical practice generally thought to work, then the question is answered with a cautious, "Yes, that does work." One example of this would be the herbalist's use of foxglove (*Digitalis purpurea*) as a heart tonic. This is something that has been done by herbalists in many parts of the world for centuries. Since an English physician discovered in the late eighteenth century that the leaf did in fact have cardiotonic properties, and since digitalis is now a standard part of the medical pharmacopoeia, many physicians would cautiously say that, "Yes, purple foxglove works as a heart tonic." The caution, of course, would come from the physician's preference that this powerful agent be prescribed by another physician in carefully measured quantities prepared by a pharmacist, rather than being given by an herbalist. However, we should keep in mind that many herbalists would have exactly the same reservations about one of their clients receiving digoxin from a physician rather than digitalis leaf gathered and prepared by an herbalist. On the matter of "understanding," I am familiar with one case in which a physician was able to successfully treat a man suffering from severe heart failure, and who also had a strong allegiance to natural remedies, only by prescribing digitalis leaf rather than the digoxin which he more frequently employed.

In many ways this theoretical method of assessing the efficacy of alternative health practices, however, is unsatisfactory. For one thing, the alternative practices in question are usually quite complex. The herbalist, for example, may consider matters of how and when to harvest an herb that are not considered by those preparing the analogous substance for the pharmacy. A variety of features of ritual and context may be seen as crucial by the herbalist and the herbalist's patient, but be simply left out of the question by the researcher making the comparison. The most common procedure is to look over the practice, eliminate everything from consideration that does not look as though it might yield a modern medical explanation (counting it as "cultural baggage") and make an assessment on the basis of what remains.

The other approach is much more difficult and expensive but, where it is feasible, it is likely to yield much more interesting results. This is what we might call the empirical (that is, based on observation) approach. In this approach one submits an alternative practice to the same kind of scientific and clinical testing by which new and promising drugs or surgical techniques originating within medicine are evaluated. This is, in fact, being done with herbal treatments from around the world, and some very valuable discoveries have been made in this way. I should perhaps emphasize *around the world*, because there seems to be a great deal more interest in systematically investigating the practices of distant peoples than of alternative practitioners who work closer to home.

However, with many alternative traditions there are major drawbacks to applying the standard investigative techniques of medical science. I have already noted that even in the case of herbs there may be a great deal left out of consideration that a traditional herbalist would have considered crucial. With other traditions it is often the case that when the investigator has finished eliminating what was taken to be "cultural baggage" there is nothing left to investigate.

Scientific research is based on experimental design and the ability to control variables. In the many traditions in which "laying on of hands" is central, for example, how can one construct a "double blind" design in which some patients really have hands laid on by a real practitioner, while other patients (the controls) don't really have hands laid on, and neither the healers nor the patients know which group is which? Or in the various traditions of prayer for healing how can the researcher treat God as a force to be manipulated and controlled? Predicting and interpreting the behavior of persons, even when they are ordinary human persons, is far more difficult than doing the same with the behavior of pharmacological agents. How much more difficult to be certain that one has understood and controlled the omniscient and omnipotent person to whom those who believe in Divine healing say that they are praying for help?

For alternative systems, then, we are faced with a dilemma. On the one hand a simple comparison of what they do with what medicine does often accomplishes nothing more than to translate some part of what the tradition does into medical language. However, empirical, scientific investigation is extremely difficult for many of these practices, as Sammons notes on burn and wart cures in chapter four. Certainly for those that are investigable, such as the herbal treatments Croom documents in his study of the Lumbee Indian culture of North Carolina in chapter eight, the effort seems worthwhile if funding can be made available. For those for which we cannot develop a plausible research design it would probably be more productive, and certainly less expensive, not to try to evaluate by standard scientific means. But I must emphasize my phrase, "if the funding is available." The practices of most alternative healing systems are at least as complex as those of modern medicine, and will be at least as expensive to submit to serious research. Considering what such research costs even in the case of new drugs and surgical techniques arising from within medical research, and therefore likely to be tailor-made for such study, adequate funding for the real study of alternative techniques will rarely be available in the near future. On the other hand, if we assume that we can answer the question, "Does it work?" in a medical sense with less than the kind of effort that we expend on new medical techniques, we are trivializing folk medicine and studying only bits and pieces of it.

What we *can* study and understand much more easily, though, is what each system says that it does, why its practitioners and clients believe that its claims are valid, and what effect the utilization of one system will have on the patients who are simultaneously using one or more others.

Conflict and Negotiation

Much of what I have already said about the coexisting health systems in the United States suggests that there exist among them varying degrees of irreconcilable differences. I consider this to be true, while at the same time granting that there are many points on which they can learn from one another, adopting and adapting specific techniques, and they may also find the bases for more collegial relationships among practitioners. This latter point is the more pleasant and easier one with which to deal. However, a serious attempt to understand and deal with such a variety of systems of thought and practice must be as much an exercise in diplomacy as in scholarship (although perhaps serious and effective diplomacy should be considered a special kind of scholarship). And effective diplomacy does not make headway by ignoring and denying real differences. As noted in the first section above, understanding must often substitute for agreement.

In those cases in which apparent conflict arises from differences in language, ideology, or inadequate data, the apparent conflicts should and can be resolved. The differences over the hospital delivery of babies and the use of birthing centers seem to be of this variety. In other cases there appear to be permanent differences that need not be taken as obstacles to effective collaboration. For example, the belief in an immortal soul that pastoral counselors and those whom they counsel generally share cannot be expected to become an official part of medical teaching in the near future. But this difference does not seriously impede the productive collaboration of medical doctors and pastoral counselors. However, there are many cases in which differences are not only firm but also are of a kind that prevents general agreements and the establishment of close, official, collegial relationships among healers. The existence of such differences, however, should not be considered a reason for the parties to such disagreements to ignore one another: quite the opposite. These are the situations in which patients are at greatest risk for being caught in the middle and in which the challenge to reach an understanding in the absence of agreement is most pressing.

In this connection I would add a cautionary note about the frequent assumption that the basic medical purpose of understanding other systems is to assimilate to conventional medicine those things that apparently "work." As I have said, some such assimilation is a sensible goal and may run in many directions (that is, not just toward medicine, but also from medicine to folk healers as is being done in the Third World by some WHO programs). But there are many other situations in which a folk healing system is simply not going about the same things—does not have the same goals—as medical doctors. Frequently, for example, when I show videotapes of religious healers to audiences that include psychiatrists I am asked "How can we teach our residents to do that?" At first the question left me completely nonplused. I realize now that there are certain aspects of the manner in which some healers present *themselves* that could be learned and used to good advantage by anyone engaged in healing. But at a more fundamental level the answer must often be "You can't teach your residents to do that, and if you more firmly grasped what was being done—you would see that that would be inappropriate." The particular case I have in mind, in which this has happened most frequently, involves a healer whose most crucial impact comes through his absolute certainty in the living presence of Christ and his certainty that physical death is a beginning and not an end. Without these two elements he would not have a healing ministry. But can we imagine these being added to a psychiatric curriculum? *Differences are as important as similarities!*

Quackery. While we are on the subject of conflict, a word needs to be said about the matter of quackery. The word "quack" is like the word "superstition." Both are used more to insult than to objectively describe. Quack means, generally, one who pretends to have medical knowledge but does not; that is, it implies the element of fraud. After years of research in this field I have no doubt that there are frauds—and many of them—taking advantage of sick people. However, most alternative healers do not pretend to have medical knowledge; they have some other sort of knowledge that they and their clients believe is relevant to health. Certainly the use of caution to protect oneself and one's family from unscrupulous and incompetent health care pretenders should be a part of everyone's concern. But this is not a concern limited to folk medicine.

We should also be careful of the criteria that we accept as discriminating between intentionally fraudulent providers and sincere (whether misguided or not) practitioners. One of the criteria that I most frequently hear suggested is whether a healer accepts money for his or her services. This is a very poor criterion indeed. For one thing, there are many incompetent individuals who are more interested in gaining notoriety, gratitude, and so forth than money. Their "charity" does not guarantee either sincerity or effectiveness. On the other hand, if we were to gauge fraudulence and assign the label "quack" on the basis of who makes the most money from a practice, many of those who have suggested this criterion would withdraw the suggestion *post haste.* There are traditions within which the acceptance of monetary repayment is simply forbidden and others in which it is not acceptable to have any set fee structure. This is one of the attractions of certain health systems. There are other systems, however, within which the practitioner is expected to be able to earn a living by his or her practice, and that fact can no more be taken as proof of fraud for a rootworker or herbalist than for a medical doctor. Furthermore, the use of terms such as quack, in the absence of specific evidence with regard to particular individuals, can only decrease the possibility of understanding and negotiation, and work to the detriment of those patients who may know for certain that the insulting label is being misapplied.

Conclusion

In conclusion, modern medicine has a great deal to offer many patients. But it takes only a little reflection to realize that it cannot offer everything that all patients need. From those forms of suffering that medicine can only partially ameliorate—and there are many of those—to the nonmedical needs of the sick—such as finding *meaning* in suffering and death—folk medicine represents the continuing response of culture to human needs. Medicine can neither assimilate all such resources nor stamp them out as unwelcome competition. For modern medicine to find its place most gracefully within community resources it must recognize the facts of cultural pluralism. And these include the fact that medicine is itself a product of culture and that it operates within culture. While it should seek to identify and reduce the risks to health that this situation occasionally presents, it cannot remove itself from the cultural sphere. Neither can it realistically aspire to providing *everything* that sick people need, even if it were to totally medicalize our entire society. The only humane course is to recognize our folk medical systems as additional community resources for dealing with sickness—resources that medicine must occasionally fight, often cooperate with, and of which we must always be aware.

Notes

1. For an excellent review of studies on this subject see Kathryn Dean, "Self-Care Responses to Illness: A Selected Review." *Social Science and Medicine* 15A (1981): 673–87.

References

Arkko, Pertti J., et al. "A Survey of Unproven Cancer Remedies and Their Users in an Outpatient Clinic for Cancer Therapy in Finland." *Social Science and Medicine* 14A (1980): 511–14.

Cassileth, Barrie R., et al. "Contemporary Unorthodox Treatments in Cancer Medicine: A Study of Patients, Treatments, and Practitioners." *Annals of Internal Medicine* 101 (1984): 105–12.

Copeland, Donna R., Yaal Silberberg, and Betty Pfefferbaum. "Attitudes and Practices of Families of Children in Treatment for Cancer: A Cross-Cultural Study." *American Journal of Pediatric Hematology and Oncology* 5 (1983): 65–71.

Dady, Peter, et al. "New Zealand Cancer Patients and Alternative Medicine." *New Zealand Journal of Medicine* 100 (1987): 110–13.

Firman, Gregory J., and Michael S. Goldstein. "The Future of Chiropractic: A Psychosocial View." *New England Journal of Medicine* 293 (1975): 639–42.

Hufford, David J. "Contemporary Folk Medicine." *Unorthodox Medicine in America.* Ed. Norman Gevitz. Baltimore: Johns Hopkins University Press, 1988. 228–64.

Lou Harris and Associates. "Health Information and the Use of Questionable Treatments: A Study of the American Public," conducted for the U.S. Department of Health and Human Services, study number 833015. September 1987.

Mooney, B. Kathleen. "Utilization of Unproven Methods of Cancer Treatment: An Investigation of Prevalence and Relevant Factors." *Dissertation Abstracts International* 46(4-A) (October 1985): 903.

Newell, S. M., et al. "Utility of the Modified Health Belief Model in Predicting Compliance with Treatment of Adult Patients with Advanced Cancer." *Psychological Reports* 59, no. 2 part 2 (1986): 783–91.

Pruyn, J. F., et al. "Cancer Patients' Personality Characteristics, Physician-Patient Communication and Adoption of the Moerman Diet." *Social Science and Medicine* 20 (1985): 841–47.

U.S. Congress, Office of Technology Assessment. *Unconventional Cancer Treatments* OTA-H-405. Washington, D.C.: U.S. Government Printing Office, September 1990.

Vogl, A. J. "It's Time to Take Chiropractors Seriously." *Medical Economics* (December 1974): 76–85.

2. Traditional Healing Today: Moving Beyond Stereotypes

Richard Blaustein

Herbal and Magical Medicine: Traditional Healing Today is an important contribution to the literature of medical folklore for a variety of reasons. First, this collection of original essays provides careful documentation of the therapeutic traditions of a long-settled and culturally diverse region which has received little serious scholarly attention until quite recently. Though the Ozarks and the southern Appalachians may loom larger in folkloristic consciousness, this book makes it clear that the lowlands of eastern North Carolina and Virginia are at least as rich in vital, ongoing traditions of folk medicine. Unlike many conventional treatments of medical folklore, the focus here is not upon listings of ailments and remedies but rather upon illuminating the role that folk medicine plays in the lives of contemporary people. Not only is this in accord with the general tendency in modern folklore scholarship toward studying the functions and values of traditional beliefs and practices in actual social contexts, but it also illustrates a strong trend in the profession toward interdisciplinary cooperation and the practical application of folkloristic knowledge and skills in a variety of educational and public service settings. From the perspective of a folklorist who is also an adjunct professor of family medicine and psychiatry, it is exciting to see other members of the profession collaborating with psychiatrists, botanists, pharmacologists, and anthropologists taking advantage of the endless fieldwork opportunities offered by their location and emphatically demonstrating that scholarship can come out of regional campuses as well as elite flagship universities. In fact, Karen Baldwin, James Kirkland, Holly Mathews, C. W. Sullivan III, and their colleagues can take credit for producing one of the very first works in the field of applied folk medicine of direct and immediate value to health care educators and their students.

This study brings home the message that folk therapies are still meaningful to many people, not only in the lowland South but throughout the modern world. Western scientific medicine is only one of many therapeutic options available to Carolinians and other contemporary Americans, and not necessarily the option of first or last resort. The belief that other medical traditions are rapidly disappearing in the wake of advances in Western medicine is a persistent, mistaken notion which could itself be called a form of folklore. As David Hufford reminds us in chapter one, ours is a medically pluralistic society.

According to Hufford, medical practitioners and educators need to come to grips with the various alternatives to official medicine that are loosely labeled as "folk medicine," and also take account of the complex beliefs, values, attitudes, protocols, and communication styles which patients *and* health care providers bring into the clinical situation. An important operating assumption, not always evident from the medical viewpoint, is that *all* health care encounters entail cross-cultural communication, even when the practitioner and patient live in the same society, speak variants of the same language, and appear to share much else in common.

Hufford exhorts us to reject stereotyped notions of folk medicine: "folk medicine is not restricted to any single region or demographically defined group. Instead, it represents a universal set of efforts to cope with illness in ways that go beyond—but do not necessarily conflict with—what modern medicine has to offer" (14–15).

Just because folk medical systems operate from differing basic assumptions does not automatically imply that they are necessarily illogical or incorrect. Indeed, as Hufford cautions us, logical consistency should not be equated with truth or efficacy. However, it is precisely when alternative medical traditions negate one another's basic assumptions, or axiomatic principles, that conflicts are most likely to emerge. Hufford presents us with the engaging picture of the medical folklorist or anthropologist seeking to mediate between the divergent cultural realities of the patient and practitioner. This is literally cultural relativism in action!

Understanding another medical culture does not, as Hufford cautions us, mean that we necessarily have to agree with it, but only that we need to take it into account, particularly as it affects effective communication between the patient and the health care provider. Something very valuable is hopefully gained as a result: the reduction of potential conflict and the possibility of dispassionate discourse and constructive negotiation. Hufford does not ask the practitioner to pretend to agree with the patient's beliefs, but rather to recognize that the patient's beliefs need to be taken into account in the prescription of a viable, effective course of treatment. Insensitivity to individual or cultural beliefs which results in noncompliance on the part of the patient underscores the connection between effective communication and successful therapy.

Alternate health care systems are extremely vigorous and persistent; they are not necessarily perpetuated by isolation, limited formal education, or poverty. Middle-class mainstream Americans, contrary to stereotyped expectations, are deeply involved in alternative therapies of various types. These alternative systems are not about to disappear anytime soon; rather, they seem to be thriving and, if anything, expanding: "It is, in fact, time to take folk medicine in general seriously," says Hufford (21).

However, this does not mean that modern scientific medicine is declining. Rather, we must understand that scientific medicine is itself a form of "alternative medicine," even though its official status is higher than that of other therapeutic systems. The medical future, as envisioned by Hufford, is characterized by "dynamic tension in an essentially pluralistic health culture" (22).

Hufford urges us to recognize that folk medical traditions are literally *systems*, sets of beliefs and practices possessing coherent, meaningful interconnections, rather than decayed, disjointed *survivals* of earlier times. Though these nonofficial therapeutic systems may not be as *complex* as modern scientific medicine, they may nonetheless possess a high level of *integration*, cognitive coherence, and consistency, which contributes to their emotional and symbolic efficacy as integrative mechanisms. However, it would be incorrect to assume that all adherents to a given therapeutic system are completely and uniformly in accord with its tenets; the individual's own beliefs, values, and attitudes should be carefully elicited, otherwise the practitioner is once again in danger of being misguided by stereotyped notions which obscure the actual complexity and diversity of modern cultural and social life in the United States and elsewhere.

The ethnographic and folkloristic studies presented in this book graphically illustrate this complexity and diversity. As Hufford asserts, most Americans take a pragmatic, eclectic approach to health care which is by no means restricted to professional Western medicine. Edward Croom's enlightening study of the herbal medical traditions of the Lumbee tribe of eastern North Carolina clearly demonstrates the complexities of modern folk medicine; the Lumbee are actually cognizant of several medical traditions, each of which is seen to have its own particular strengths and weaknesses. Croom's treatment of herbalism is unusually valuable because he has gone to great lengths to establish not only the positive, curative properties of the medical plants used by the Lumbee, but also problems of cumulative toxicity which could occur as a result of their continual, unregulated use. Like the Lumbee, most of us are actually self-maintainers who will make use of any form of health care we deem to be effective; it is estimated that perhaps only one out of ten incidents of illness or injury ever receives the attention of medical practitioners. Folk medical beliefs and practices are by no means confined to the poor, the isolated, or the uneducated as C. W. Sullivan III shows in chapter nine. Though many ethnomedical beliefs and practices are based on premises which violate the canons of conventional biomedicine, they cannot all be simply dismissed as superstition, pseudoscience, or quackery. Linda Camino's article on spiritual heart disease (chapter seven) shows the importance of understanding how the basic premises expressed within a medical belief system serve to determine how distress is interpreted by the individual and how it is presented to others. Psychosomatic distress still continues to frustrate the diagnostic efforts of professionally trained physicians, largely due to cultural and conceptual gaps between patient and practitioner. However, as the contributions by physicians in this volume indicate, progressive medical practitioners and researchers recognize that the serious study of folk medicine can lead to a better understanding of human health and healing in general.

While no single therapeutic system is totally efficacious, the diverse forms of folk medicine still flourishing in the modern world have survived because they do succeed in many cases in providing relief from distress and stimulating the integrative capacities of the human mind and body, raising fundamental and intriguing questions concerning symbolic communication and the healing process. As the eminent medical anthropologist Arthur Kleinman has written, "For researchers in clinical medicine, healing is an embarrassing word. It exposes the archaic roots of medicine and psychiatry which are usually buried under the biomedical facade of modern health care. . . . [I]t raises questions which deal with human values and meanings that are not easily reduced to technical questions which can be answered with simple biological explanations" (Kleinman and Sung 7). While Western scientific medicine has been highly successful in developing effective techniques for dealing with disease or biophysical trauma, Kleinman and others have noted that it has been considerably less successful in helping patients come to terms with psychosocial trauma or illness.

Though lacking the formal training and awesome armamentarium of the modern scientifically trained physician, traditional healers often display effective practical knowledge of the psychological and emotional needs of their patients, which leads to successful healing on various levels. As the structural anthropologist Claude Lévi-Strauss has suggested, the folk healer gives the patient "a *language*, by means of which unexpressed, and otherwise unexpressible, psychic states can be immediately expressed. And it is the transition to this verbal expression—at the same time making it possible to undergo in an orderly and intelligible form a real experience that would otherwise be chaotic and inexpressible—which induces the release of the physiological process" (198). More simply put, by locating and identifying sources of distress within a culturally and socially meaningful context, the healer imposes order, definition, and structure upon disintegrative experiences, connecting with the patient with integrative resources that make distress psychologically manageable, promoting physical as well as emotional healing.

Just how this primordial process of mind-body interplay operates is a subject of intense scientific interest and speculation. Indeed, the father of semiotics, Thomas Sebeok, calls the problem of the conversion of symbolic information into metabolic responses "the ultimate enigma." To quote Sebeok, "As Jacob von Uexkull might have phrased it, how are semiotic strings—verbal or nonverbal—emanating from the organism's *Umwelt,* transmuted into beneficial or harmful effects in the body's *Innenwelt?* Or to adapt Lévi-Strauss' opposition, how are subjective states—let us call them 'Culture'—transformed into 'Nature'?" (201).

This ultimate enigma is pursued in chapters three and four by James Kirkland and Robert Sammons, dealing with magico-religious healing of burns and warts and possible connections with clinical hypnosis. Sammons supports Kirkland's observation that folk healers believe that they can alleviate pain and also cause burns to heal without disfiguring scars. There is impressive medical literature demonstrating the efficacy of hypnotism in reducing the physical as well as the psychological trauma of severe burns. It appears that hypnotism suppresses the body's natural inflammatory response to burns, which normally results in scarification, and otherwise permits rapid restoration of healthy tissue structure; warts are cured by the restriction of blood flow to surrounding tissue and also possibly by the symbolically induced secretion of antiviral substances. Warts seem to be especially susceptible to the power of suggestion, and it has long been observed that a wide variety of curative rituals will cause them to disappear. In a state of heightened suggestibility (whatever that might exactly be), symbolically mediated messages are communicated directly to those sections of the brain that govern basic integrative responses without the usual cognitive dissonance and emotional feedback which characterizes normal waking consciousness. Conversely, when the individual is overwhelmed by uncontrolled physical or psychological trauma, contradictory messages may result in the breakdown of metabolic homeostasis and actually result, as Walter B. Cannon stated in his classic article on "Voodoo Death" (1943), in disintegration and dissolution unless counteracting integrative resources can be provided.

Another pair of companion pieces (chapters five and six) by anthropologist Holly Mathews and clinical physician Peter Lichstein, dealing with the eclectic tradition of sorcery and magical healing known as "rootwork," focus on reintegration of the sick or hexed person into a coherent, meaningful social network. All cultural belief systems about illness provide cognitive structure that helps "individuals and communities cope with the anxieties and uncertainties of illness." The patient asks the doctor "to help bring order to the chaos of illness" (100). Every culture provides the individuals who have internalized it with a shared frame of reference consisting of sets of basic assumptions through which we interpret and make sense out of the experiential universe. These include axiomatic concepts of the origin and fundamental nature of the mind and body which, in turn, determine concepts of the causation and classification of disease that are expressed in diagnostic and therapeutic systems. As Lichstein and Mathews concur, cultural conflict can easily arise when patients confront medical practitioners who are ignorant of their cultural beliefs and social expectations regarding interpersonal communication of distress—especially when the purported source of distress falls outside of the practitioner's notions of what is real and possible, as in the case of illnesses believed to be magically induced by rootwork. On a very practical level it is clear that the practitioner's ability to understand the patient's frame of reference (as reflected in the presentation and interpretation of symptoms) plays a critical role in ensuring compliance to an appropriate therapeutic regimen and initiating successful healing. One reason why alternative therapeutic systems are so vital in the modern world is precisely because so many people are frustrated by the inability of mechanistic biomedicine to provide intellectually meaningful and emotionally satisfying explanations and interpretations and effectively alleviate psychological trauma. On the other hand, folk healers are often capable of satisfying their patients' needs for meaningfulness and connectedness and thereby activating symbolically induced healing through the power of suggestion or faith or belief.

Though we are still far from precise knowledge of the neurochemical hierarchies responsible for symbolically induced healing, it would appear that some of our most important integrative resources are social support and traditional expressive culture. The effective healer utilizes various forms of symbolic expression characterized by a high degree of redundancy and predictability which reduce cognitive and emotional distress, lending support to Karen Baldwin's contention in chapter ten that the formal and aesthetic features of healing charms and rituals contribute to their therapeutic value. Rhythm, meter, balance, and symmetry may literally cut through the subjective chaos of unmediated distress and restore the control of the symbol-generating cerebral cortex over the hypothalamus and limbic system.

The emotional value which the patient invests in a given mode of treatment and a particular practitioner has a great deal to do with the success or failure of any therapeutic regimen; Kleinman and Sung contend that "the question of healing makes it apparent that much of clinical science can only be approached from the perspective of social science" (7). Symbolically induced healing is fundamentally a social phenomenon; confidence in the practitioner and belief in the efficacy of the proposed treatment is significantly responsible for cueing the healing process. As Robert Ornstein and David Sobel assert in *The Healing Brain,* "Obviously there are limits to the ability to be able to control bodily functions through mental means. Yet the impact of intangibles like words and symbols, when leveraged through a brain whose major form of exchange is such thoughts, can be powerful. Words can be scalpels. They can generate thoughts, feelings and beliefs in our brain which can be communicated to the cells of our body and even to the chemicals within cells" (103–4). Medical anthropologist Daniel Moerman hypothesizes that "the personality of the physician and the enthusiasm with which he embraces his procedures can create a symbolic field which, perceived by the patient, can influence him to trigger autonomous healing mechanisms" (263–64). The effectiveness of placebos, clinical hypnosis, and various types of folk therapy all depend upon the establishment of rapport between practitioner and patient in which confusion, mistrust, and anxiety are minimized, resulting in a wide variety of specific integrative responses including the production of endorphins (pain suppressors), interferons (antiviral agents) and steroids (counterinflammatory agents). According to the psychological anthropologist Francis L. K. Hsu, contact with significant others is essential to the individual's sense of psychological and emotional well-being; the weakening or loss of meaning-filled social relationships is profoundly stressful. A substantial body of medical literature supports the thesis that the breakdown of crucial social relationships leads to physiological deterioration and disintegration. Emotional stress can suppress the immune system, cause blood pressure to rise, send conflicting messages to the heart which cause it to tear itself apart, and otherwise devastate an organism made vulnerable by grief, despair, or inexpressible hostility. Here again the insights of Claude Lévi-Strauss into the psychological and social dynamics of the healing relationship are particularly relevant: "The patient is all passivity and self-alienation, just as inexpressibility is the disease of the mind. The sorcerer is activity and self-projection, just as affectivity is the source of symbolism. The cure interrelates these opposite poles, facilitating the transition from one to the other, and demonstrates, within a total experience, the coherence of the psychic universe, itself a projection of the social universe" (182).

Whether assessing the implications of archaic yet effective techniques employed by folk healers or recent discoveries in the still evolving field of psychoneuroimmunology, modern medicine must come to terms with the whole person as a social, cultural, and spiritual being, rather than treating the body as a senseless automaton and the mind as a meaningless illusion. The creative collaboration here between academic researchers and clinical practitioners shows that a more humane and culturally sensitive approach to healing is emerging which is capable of appreciating the accumulated wisdom of folk healers along with the brilliant insights of twentieth-century medical pioneers like Hans Selye and René Dubos, who urged his fellow physicians to restore the human element to the therapeutic equation: "Ever since the 17th century, medical science has been shaped largely by Cartesian analytical philosophy. Its ideal is to subdivide every anatomic structure, physiological function, and biochemical process into smaller and smaller subunits so that each can be studied in greater and greater detail. . . . [T]o a large extent, all systems of medicine except those based on Western science derive from an emphasis on the integration of the body, mind and environment" (Dubos 30–31). Dubos believed that the future progress of Western medical science depended upon its ability to recognize the limitations of its own historical past and to realize once again the fundamental interdependence of mind and body, individual and society, humanity and the natural world. The publication of *Herbal and Magical Medicine: Traditional Healing Today* is an important practical step in that direction; hopefully it will provide a model for further cooperation between scholars, researchers, and practitioners who have devoted themselves to alleviating suffering and improving the human condition.

References

Dubos, René. "Health and Creative Adaptation." *The Nation's Health.* Ed. Philip R. Lee, Carroll L. Estes, and Nancy B. Ramsay. 2d ed. San Francisco: Boyd and Fraser, 1984. 25–32.

Kleinman, Arthur, and Lilias H. Sung. "Why Do Indigenous Practitioners Successfully Heal?" *Social Science and Medicine* 13B (1979): 7–26.

Levi-Strauss, Claude. *Structural Anthropology.* New York: Basic, 1963.

Moerman, Daniel E. "Edible Symbols: The Effectiveness of Placebos." Sebeok and Rosenthal. 256–67.

Ornstein, Robert, and David Sobel. *The Healing Brain.* New York: Simon and Schuster, 1987.

Sebeok, Thomas. "The Ultimate Enigma of 'Clever Hans': The Union of Nature and Culture." Sebeok and Rosenthal. 199–205.

Sebeok, Thomas, and Robert Rosenthal, eds. *The Clever Hans Phenomenon: Communication with Horses, Whales, Apes, and People.* New York: Annals of the New York Academy of Science, 1982.

3. Talking Fire out of Burns:

A Magico-Religious Healing Tradition

James Kirkland

It happens suddenly, unexpectedly, with the flaring of a grease fire, with a careless step into a bed of low-burning coals, with the ignition of excess gasoline spilling over the hot metallic surface of a tractor, or with something as commonplace as an overturned cup of coffee. Whatever the cause, however minor or serious the burn, the pain is always intense—the desire for relief immediate and insistent. At such a time, many people call a physician or rush to the emergency room of the nearest hospital; others seek aid from another source—from community healers who possess the power to "talk out fire."

Theirs is an ancient art—a form of magico-religious healing that has been traced back at least as far as the Middle Ages and documented in the medical lore of Europe and various sections of the United States, including the Ozarks, Louisiana, Indiana, Illinois, Pennsylvania, Michigan, and parts of the Southeast. The published record is by no means complete, however, for there are regions which have not yet been investigated and issues that have not yet been addressed in any systematic way. The objective of this study is to explore some of the most important aspects of the burn-healing tradition of one such area—the coastal plains of North Carolina—and, in the process, to dispel some of the misconceptions disseminated in published works.

One of the few reliable, scholarly resources is the sixth volume of *The Frank C. Brown Collection of North Carolina Folklore, Popular Beliefs and Superstitions from North Carolina,* which includes several field-collected items from North Carolina informants (all from central and western counties) together with extensive annotations and comparative notes by Wayland Hand. Other publications dealing with the subject consist mainly of scattered notes and source studies; patronizing commentaries like Ina Forbus's "Orange County Home Cures" and Charles Burgin's "The Extraction of Pain from Burns"; and articles such as James Rogers's "Talking Fire out of Burns," in which the author makes sweeping generalizations about healers, patients, treatment procedures, and provenience on the basis of what he himself refers to as "a few scattered and undetailed accounts" (46). More to the point is Michael Owen Jones's brief but insightful discussion of faith healing in a more broadly focused article entitled "Toward an Understanding of Folk Medical Beliefs in North Carolina"; but since he deals exclusively with the materials in the *Brown Collection,* neither this work nor the previously mentioned sources include any accounts from informants in the state's eastern counties, where my own research shows there is a thriving magico-religious healing tradition.[1]

Rather than attempting to document the beliefs and practices of all the informants I have surveyed during the past twelve years, I have focused here on a representative group of healers from four eastern North Carolina counties. Representing Pitt County is Stella Buck, a white practitioner in her early seventies. From Lenoir County come two of the most active burn healers in the coastal plains area, Kathleen Johnson and Walter King, both caucasians in their late fifties. Wilson County also has an extensive burn-healing tradition, which has been carried on for decades by Vira Turnage Blackmon, a white informant in her early sixties, and her eighty-year-old sister Roena Turnage Hockaday. The three remaining informants—Genevieve Gray, a black practitioner in her late fifties; Arthur Banks, a black healer of approximately the same age; and Iney Mae Joyner, a white woman in her early seventies—are all residents of Edgecombe County.[2]

At the heart of all the cures used by burn healers is a charm through which the practitioner summons divine powers to the aid of the sufferer. Some healers, such as Genevieve Gray of Sharpsburg and Arthur Banks of Rocky Mount, invoke the name of the deity in concentrated, one-verse formulas like "God the Father, God the Son" or "God forgot it." Others, such as Stella Buck, a lifelong resident of the town of Blackjack, quote directly from the Bible such verses as Matthew 28:18–20:

> And Jesus . . . spake unto them, saying,
> All power is given unto me in heaven and in earth.

> Go ye, therefore, and teach all nations, baptizing them in the name of the Father, and of the Son, and of the Holy Ghost:
>
> Teaching them to observe all things whatsoever I have commanded you: and, lo, I am with you alway, even unto the end of the world.

More typical is the use of a short, symbolically charged verse dramatizing the conquest of Frost over Fire. In one version, related to me by Iney Mae Joyner of Rocky Mount,

> There came three angels from the West,
> Three angels of the best,
> Three angels of God.
> Go away fire and come frost.

In another, Roena Turnage Hockaday of Bentonville gives an even more vivid account of the conflict:

> I saw six angels coming from the North
> Three had fire, three had frost.
> Go out fire; come in frost.
> through the name of the Lord, the Son,
> and the Holy Ghost.

An unusual variant of the latter verse was communicated to me by the informant's sister, Vira Turnage Blackmon, who substitutes two Indians for six angels, but with the same symbolic outcome:

> I saw two Indians from the North
> One had fire, the other had frost.
> Out fire; in frost.
> Son of God and Holy Ghost.

In yet another charm which the healer—Kathleen Johnson of Deep Run—told me only on the condition that I not publicly reveal the exact words, it is the Mother of God who combats the fire and performs the ritual exorcism.

I have not as yet found any exact parallels to the first two charms, though verses of comparable length are cited in Thomas Forbes's "Verbal Charms in British Folk Medicine," but most of the other charms cited here have numerous analogues. Most obvious are the similarities between the verse formulas used by Iney Mae Joyner, Roena Hockaday, and Vira Blackmon, and the following charms collected from informants in western North Carolina, northeastern Georgia, and the Ozarks, respectively:

> There came two angels from the north
> One brought fire; and one brought frost
> Go out fire and come in frost. (Stroup 266)

> Thair came an angel
> from the East bringing
> frost and fire. In frost out
> fire. In the name of
> the father the Son and
> of the Holy Goost. (Wigginton 367)

> Two little angels came from
> Heaven, one brought fire and the
> other brought frost, go out fire
> and come in frost. (Randolph 122)

Kathleen Johnson's formulaic address to the Virgin Mary is also akin to charms collected from informants in other areas, such as this verse from Emma Gertrude White's "Folk Medicine among Pennsylvania Germans":

> The blessed Virgin went over the land.
> What does she carry in her hand?
> A fire-brand.
> Eat not in thee. Eat not farther around.
> In the name of the Father, and of the Son,
> And of the Holy Ghost. (78)

Whatever verses the healer might use, only rarely are the words comprehensible to the patient or anyone else who might be present. The one exception among my informants is Stella Buck, who reads aloud from the Bible. All the others repeat the words silently or mumble the verse in such garbled tones that no one can understand it. As Walter King, a practitioner from Deep Run, explains, "It doesn't matter who's there—if you were right there in the room, you couldn't tell what I was saying." Similar procedures are cited in most of the published accounts from North Carolina and elsewhere, though threefold repetition of the charm, which has been frequently noted by other collectors, is not common among my informants, who say that the number of repetitions varies, depending upon the severity of the burn.

Another important aspect of the curative process is the use of homeopathic or contagious magic as an accompaniment to the secret incantation. Several of my informants—Stella Buck, Genevieve Gray, and Arthur Banks—"draw out" the fire by moving their fingers or hand in a circular or lateral pattern over the wound without actually touching it. Others seek to transmit the healing power of the Holy Spirit directly to the wound by rubbing and/or blowing on it. According to Kathleen Johnson, "you put your hand where the burn is—hold it still if the burn is small; if not, you rub it." In like manner, Vira Blackmon puts "her fingers over the top of the burned place" before reciting her charm. Her sister Roena follows a more involved procedure, which she explains in this way: "If a person gets burned a lot of them comes here to me for me to talk the fire out and I talk and rub it and blow it." In these respects, their approach resembles that of practitioners such as the Pennsylvania powwower whose treatment procedure is described in S. P. Bayard's "Witchcraft, Magic and Spirits on the Border of Pennsylvania and West Virginia":

> To "blow the fire out of a
> burn," rub your forefinger about
> the edge of the burn three times.
> At each rub, say the charm.

Less widespread, apparently, is a supplemental treatment used by many eastern North Carolina practitioners, who apply various substances to the surface of the burn while performing their magical rites. Vira Blackmon, who has been talking out fire for the people of Bentonville ever since she was a child, gently applies alcohol to the wound. "Store liquor will do," she told me, "but pure alcohol is better if you can get it." Genevieve Gray, Stella Buck, and others prefer an ointment, though they don't seem particular about what kind. As the latter puts it, "Lord, honey, it don't matter what kind; you just grease a collard leaf and put it on. That's the best thing to do because it don't stick to the skin like cloth does." I have also been told that toothpaste, axle grease, homemade lard, and even spit work well as pain-killing agents.

A few healers, such as Walter King, combine magical elements and medicinal substances with other rituals. He begins with a ritual test of faith, asking "Do you believe in the Bible?" a question that he says is always answered in the affirmative. Then he proceeds with the cure, which he effects by mumbling a charm "quoted from Scripture" while gently blowing on the wound. If he is treating someone in his own home, he keeps toothpaste nearby so that he can apply it whenever necessary to soothe the pain while he performs the more significant elements of the cure; if someone goes to him at work, he relies entirely on the faith healing rites. In either case, he observes two taboos. The first is one that I have not seen or heard anywhere else: "I'm not supposed to talk the fire out with my cap on or my hat," he told me. "I can't say much more about it except that you take your cap or hat off in church, don't you?" The second prohibition governs the actions of the patient or, if the burn victim is a child, the behavior of the parents: "You're not supposed to thank me or say 'How much do we owe you?' Mostly them that says 'We thank you, what do we owe you?' has to come back—you're supposed to walk right on out and not say anything."

The latter belief is adhered to by only two other practitioners I am familiar with—Genevieve Gray and Arthur Banks—but there is another kind of taboo that is commonly observed in all areas where the tradition exists, one that governs the transmission of the gift. With few exceptions, healers believe that the secret may be passed only between persons of the opposite sex. All but one of the practitioners I have interviewed said that they had been taught how to "talk out fire" by someone of the opposite sex and that they could not share it except under the same conditions. Breaking the taboo would mean that they and, according to the belief of some informants, the person who taught them the secret would lose the power.

There are exceptions, however. Stella Buck, for example, will communicate her knowledge to persons of either sex, and I have talked with one female practitioner who acquired the gift directly from her grandmother. Other beliefs concerning the transmission process are also worth noting. Kathleen Johnson stipulates that the secret must not be transmitted from one family member to another, even if the two people are of the opposite sex. Arthur Banks adheres to the tradition of cross-sex transmission but he believes that any woman other than a member of his own household can be told the secret. Thus he has communicated it to his daughter who is married and lives a few houses away but will not teach his wife how to "talk out fire" as long as they are living together. Walter King, following yet another custom, requires not only that the prospective recipient be a woman but that she be able to memorize the charm the first and only time he repeats it. A comparable practice is mentioned in *Ozark Superstitions*, where Vance Randolph describes a power doctor who refused to repeat the charm more than three times on the grounds that anyone who couldn't learn it under those circumstances wasn't qualified to perform the cure.

Some burn healers also limit the number of people with whom they will share the secret, but there are a great many others—including all of the practitioners that I have interviewed—who set no restrictions at all, a fact that Rogers seems unaware of when he asserts, categorically, that "The 'power' may be given to three people, all of whom must be sexual opposites of the practitioner. When the third and final person is told, the original 'fire doctor' loses the ability to administer the cure" (49).

One must also be cautious in generalizing about the healers themselves and the people they treat. For neither can be fitted to a single prototype or defined in terms of stereotypes based on what Don Yoder, in another context refers to as "Enlightenment labels of 'superstition' and 'quack medicine'" that reduce all folk medicine to a mere "'curiosity show' of peasant credulity" (211).

The burn healers surveyed in this study are in many respects a heterogeneous group composed of whites and blacks, men as well as women—people who perform different jobs, belong to different religious denominations, and speak in different dialects. Yet they share certain qualities that make them well-known and respected members of their communities. Unlike such charismatic, egocentric faith healers as the fabled Jim Gallagher, whom Michael Owen Jones profiles in his monograph *Why Faith Healing?*, they are deeply religious, self-effacing people who regard themselves not as the absolute possessors of the power to heal but as intermediaries between God and their fellow human beings. They express this conviction in different words, but the following statement by Stella Buck is representative: "The Lord does the work; I don't have a bit of any strength in the world. It's all in God." They are also very compassionate people, who express their concern for others through both words and actions. Vira Blackmon speaks for all the healers I have interviewed when she explains, "I just do it to help out if I can. I think if anybody's hurt or needs help like that I'm just glad if I can be of assistance to them." Furthermore, she and others like her open their doors to all who seek their help, they go into other people's homes when called upon for assistance, and—unlike their commercialized counterparts, the highway healers who advertise their services under banners like "Sister Serena," "Mother Divine," and "Madam Lorainne" or the pray-for-pay orators of the radio and TV ministry—they charge no fees. The numerous case histories they relate also reveal another common character trait, the ability to empathize with their patients. Nowhere is this sympathetic response more apparent than in Walter King's description of the pain and discomfort he inflicts upon himself in order to draw the fire out of someone else:

> A little boy pulled over a coffee pot, and his grandmother came to the store and said, "Walter, come—and come now. The baby is burnt bad. . . ." I got there and he was burnt awful bad. A child's skin is tenderer than mine or yours. . . . And I went ahead, and he squalled, which they will. You put your lips—I've had my lips to crack open from it—you put your lips close to it and you go over the burnt place, and you start it, and you keep working around, working around, until you get back where you started. I could see the water running out of him, just like sweat. . . . I had to stop several times and dry my lips; your lips will crack open if you don't use vaseline or chapstick or something.

Testimonials of this kind are indicative, too, of the practitioners' conceptions of the potency of the cure and its results. Although Thomas Forbes, Elizabeth Brandon, and others have concluded that the main purpose of the treatment is to alleviate pain, all but one of the practitioners in my survey believe that by drawing the fire out of the wound they not only relieve the victim's suffering but also make it possible for the wound to heal without blistering or scarring.

In the previously mentioned case the child stopped crying shortly after the treatment, and—according to Walter King—the burns healed without any trace of a scar. Similar results are cited by other healers, among them Kathleen Johnson, who says that she once treated her granddaughter for a burn that was initially very painful but stopped hurting within an hour after the cure was performed and "didn't scar bad." Even more striking is Stella Buck's account of an incident that is reminiscent of the well-known long-distance cure reported by Richard Dorson in *Bloodstoppers and Bearwalkers:*

> There was a man that got burned real bad. . . . He had some brush around his yard, so he got some gas and put it on this trash to start the fire and the wind shifted and blowed that fire right back on him. He was burnt real bad. So he called me and said, "Miss Stella I'm burned and I'd like to get to you now but I ain't got no way." And I says, "Well, I can't get to you either but I'll get to you as soon as I can if I can get someone to carry me." So I waited for a few minutes and started talking to the Lord and by the time I got there you know his pain wasn't even hurting him. The Lord had done touched his body before I could even get there.

It does not necessarily follow, however, that folk burn healers consider their practices incompatible with more conventional forms of health care. On the contrary, all the healers I am familiar with have regular doctors, whom they consult for most ailments, and are quick to praise physicians who display skill and concern. Moreover, burn doctors often seem able to recognize when a wound is serious enough to require professional medical attention. As Walter King told the mother of a child he had just treated, "If infection starts, you've got to use antibiotics. Take her to your family doctor; it's burned deeper than you think it is."

The people who seek this form of alternative medical care for themselves or their families are as diversified as the healers themselves. Even in the relatively small group of patients that I have interviewed, there are farmers, truck drivers, factory workers, college students, university professors, ministers, pharmacists, and even a member of the board of directors of a large county hospital. Whatever their occupation, age, race, or religion, a remarkably large number of people throughout eastern North Carolina consult burn healers instead of, or in addition to, licensed physicians.

Kathleen Johnson, for example, claims to have talked the fire out of more than 300 people in the 15 years or so that she has known how to perform the cure; and most of the others—though less specific about numbers—describe their healing activities as "steady" or "frequent." Just how frequently and under what circumstances they are called upon to work their beneficent magic is evident from this succession of case histories related by Vira Blackmon:

> I was working in the candy plant one time and a boy said that he didn't believe in talking out fire. In about two to three hours, hot water got spilled in his shoes and all and he came running to me and . . . he didn't even have to go to the doctor. From then on, he said he'd never say he didn't believe in talking out fire.
>
> I've had boys, people to come from all over the community; one particular boy had got burned fixing a tractor and oh, he had been to the doctor but he came for me to talk out the fire.
>
> And then, I've had people to burn their hands. They'd be in other occupations that would come and I'd talk the fire out.
>
> I'd be cooking supper you know or breakfast and people would get burned with hot grease or something and they'd take off over here just as soon as it happened to have the fire talked out.
>
> At the plant the other day, I was coming out of work and this supervisor stopped and called me—she had burned her hand two days

> before then—and I talked the fire out. In two days I asked her how was it and she said "almost well."

Although patients sometimes travel great distances to reach folk practitioners such as Vira Blackmon, most live in the healers' own communities and know their benefactors personally as a result of their frequent contact with one another through their jobs, church affiliations, and civic or recreational activities. Even if a prospective patient were not personally acquainted with the healer, the former could scarcely avoid hearing about this individual's accomplishments because narratives like the ones cited throughout this study circulate throughout the community via an informal but efficient medical information and referral system.

A thorough study of this communications network is beyond the scope of this essay (for additional information about this process, see my "Traditional Medical Information Systems in Deep Run, North Carolina"), but the following narrative offers a striking example of how patients and practitioners are sometimes brought together and what goes through the minds of burn victims before, during, and after the treatment. The informant is Deborah Battle, a young black woman who at the time of our interview was a student at Edgecombe Technical College; her story concerns an event that had occurred several years earlier when she had an unanticipated meeting with Arthur Banks:

> I was cooking . . . and there was some hot oil, and it was bubbling hot all over my face, and all my jaw here was burned and I ran to my mother's house. She took me to this man and he told me to sit down and then he told me whenever he got through don't say "thank you" or it won't work. And he took his hand and went like this over the burn. He never said anything, he was just steadily moving his mouth. And as he moved his hand down I could feel the heat vanishing. . . . It never did leave any scars, either.

Why this burn victim—like so many others—felt her pain diminish almost the instant the healer began the ritual or why her face and neck bore no trace of a scar are questions that must be left to experts in other fields. But the accounts of patients, practitioners, and others involved either directly or indirectly with the tradition do lead to at least one indisputable conclusion: that there is, indeed, a magico-religious burn-healing tradition in eastern North Carolina—a tradition of great magnitude and vitality—that deserves the same degree of scholarly attention accorded the similar practices of Ozark power doctors, Louisiana traiteurs, and Pennsylvania German powwowers. Only by that means can we truly hope to understand the nature and functions of this folk healing art or comprehend why people sometimes drive past modern medical centers on their way to Deep Run or Sharpsburg or wherever else there are individuals who know how to "talk out fire."

Notes

1. A great deal of the data cited in this essay were collected during the late 1970s and early 1980s with the support of a research grant from East Carolina University, but the findings reported here are by no means limited to that time period. On the contrary, subsequent fieldwork and archive research indicate that the tradition continues to flourish in communities throughout eastern North Carolina, manifesting itself in the same kinds of beliefs and practices described by informants who participated in the original survey.

2. The biographical information included here pertains to the informants' age, residence, occupation, and the like at the time each of them was interviewed.

References

Bayard, S. P. "Witchcraft, Magic and Spirits on the Border of Pennsylvania and West Virginia." *Journal of American Folklore* 41 (1928): 47–59.

Brandon, Elizabeth. "Folk Medicine in French Louisiana." *American Folk Medicine: A Symposium.* Ed. Wayland D. Hand. Berkeley: University of California Press, 1976. 215–34.

Burgin, Charles E. "The Extraction of Pain from Burns." *North Carolina Folklore* 8 (1960): 17–18.

Dorson, Richard. *Bloodstoppers and Bearwalkers.* Cambridge, Mass.: Harvard University Press, 1952.

Forbes, Thomas. "Verbal Charms in British Folk Medicine." *Proceedings of the American Philosophical Society* 115.4 (1971): 293–316.

Forbus, Ina B. "Orange County Home Cures." *North Carolina Folklore* 8 (1960): 12–16.

Hand, Wayland D., ed. *Popular Beliefs and Superstitions from North Carolina.* Vol. 6 of *The Frank C. Brown Collection of North Carolina Folklore.* Durham, N.C.: Duke University Press, 1961.

Jones, Michael Owen. "Toward an Understanding of Folk Medical Beliefs in North Carolina." *North Carolina Folklore Journal* 30 (1982): 43–51.

Kirkland, James W. "Traditional Medical Information Systems in Deep Run, North Carolina." *North Carolina Folklore Journal* 30 (1982): 43–51.

Randolph, Vance. *Ozark Superstitions.* New York: Dover, 1964.

Rogers, James. "Talking Fire out of Burns." *North Carolina Folklore* 16 (1968): 46–52.

Stroup, Thomas. "A Charm from North Carolina and *The Merchant of Venice,* II, vii, 75." *Journal of American Folklore* 49 (1936): 266.

White, Emma Gertrude. "Folk Medicine among Pennsylvania Germans." *Journal of American Folklore* 10 (1897): 78–80.

Wigginton, Eliot, ed. "Faith Healing." *The Foxfire Book.* New York: Doubleday, 1971. 348–68.

Yoder, Don. "Folk Medicine." *Folklore and Folklife.* Ed. Richard Dorson. Chicago: University of Chicago Press, 1972. 191–215.

4. Parallels Between Magico-Religious Healing and Clinical Hypnosis Therapy

Robert Sammons

My introduction to folk healing came through a rather embarrassing story that was told about my father. After his graduation from a prestigious southern medical school, my father went to visit his in-laws on their farm in Tennessee. During this particular visit a goat man that my grandfather had befriended in the past stopped to pay his respects at my grandfather's farm. Goat men, who would surely receive a psychiatric diagnosis today, were vagabonds who traveled in small, mule-drawn wagons containing all their worldly possessions and were usually escorted by a few goats. Ostracized by most of society at that time, goat men also scared other people because of their unconventional behavior and beliefs concerning folk healing. On shaking hands with my father, the goat man noticed a wart on my father's finger and began to rub it with a copper penny, saying that it would be gone in five days. Although medical science at that time did not know what caused warts, the acceptable procedure for wart removal taught in medical school did not include rubbing it with a penny. My father took the good-natured rubbing in stride, confident that five days later he would have the last laugh. Much to his chagrin, the wart was gone in five days.

Folk medicine has been the predominant form of medicine practiced across time and is still the majority form of medicine practiced in the world today. Many of those who read this book will have a strong curiosity about folk medicine and folk cures. Most readers will have been raised in an era in which scientific medicine has been increasingly effective, but many have witnessed a folk cure in the past, have heard a story like the one told about my father, or have read descriptions of cures like those cited in other chapters of this book. In this day of high technology, some may snicker and relegate to pure superstition the practice of root or folk medicine. When our most sophisticated burn units find it difficult to achieve success with a burned patient, it is tempting to trivialize the less technical and seemingly unsophisticated folk practices. When folk medicine is discussed seriously, two issues are generally raised: whether or not the folk practices work and, if they work, what mechanism produces their effect.

Because folk practices occur in the community rather than in a university setting, good research with tight experimental design is not available to evaluate their efficacy. Sufficient anecdotal evidence does exist, however, to suggest that many folk cures do produce their anticipated result. Folk cures are influenced by laws of behavior and function differently from general superstitions. For example, if a person wears a lucky rabbit's foot and waits for something to happen, with sufficient passage of time some event will occur that the person can interpret as being fortunate and, therefore, give credit to the rabbit's foot. Under this condition neither the time course nor the specific event is predicted. In folk cures, on the other hand, a specific outcome is anticipated and the time interval is certainly noted. In the example of a burned person going to a folk healer who talks fire out of burns, the goal is relief from pain and the time interval is expected to be fairly short. Thus, folk healers are given an empirical test each time someone comes to see them. If specific relief is not given within a reasonable time period, the folk healer will lose his or her practice. Thus, the laws of learning apply to folk healing as they do to other aspects of our behavior. Behaviors that are reinforced continue, while those that aren't reinforced fade. The fact that traditional medicine has persisted in a culture with advanced medical technology suggests that there has been some level of efficacy in the folk treatment.

If one accepts the hypothesis that folk healing has persisted because of its effectiveness in certain areas, the next question is how does it work? One answer is that the procedures simply work by the magico-religious explanation given by the folk healers. But such an hypothesis is difficult to accept, given our extensive knowledge of biochemistry and pathophysiology. A more plausible explanation is that many folk cures, particularly those for burns and warts, are effected through hypnotic suggestions—a theory that provides a bridge between folk medicine and current scientific medical knowledge.

Though some regard hypnosis as nothing more than parlor entertainment, it is in fact a powerful medical instrument. To analyze the relationship between hypnosis and folk cures, one must first understand a few basic facts about hypnosis. Hypnosis may best be thought of as a state of heightened cognitive arousal or suggestion where the body is able to do things it is not normally able to do. For example, if you offer a person $3,000 to lift a car or tractor, most would be unable to do that. But we are all familiar with reports of women in times of emergency lifting cars off their children or tractors off their husbands. In a similar way, it is difficult for most of us to stretch out between two chairs with our heads resting on one chair and feet on the other, with no support in between, much less sustaining any weight on our abdomens. But one of the more popular demonstrations by night club hypnotists is to stretch hypnotized subjects between two chairs with their heads on one end and heels on the other and no support in the middle. An especially brazen hypnotist may even stand on a person's stomach or break rocks there with a sledgehammer while the hypnotized subject is suspended between two chairs. Although hypnosis cannot make the body do something that isn't possible, hypnosis can allow the body to do things it is not normally able to do.

Pain is another good example of a normal body response that can sometimes be interrupted, but generally without our control. Most of us have had experiences in which we have sustained an injury during a time of excitement, such as scoring a touchdown or chasing after a child in danger, but felt no pain until after the excitement or anxiety had subsided. In a similar way, hypnoanesthesia has been used to block pain. This method has proven to be so effective that it has been used as the sole anesthesia in a caesarean section. Thus, we have another example of hypnosis enabling the body to engage in a process that it is capable of doing, but not under normal motivational circumstances.

The thesis proposed in this essay is that two specific forms of folk healing, "talking fire out of burns" and removing warts, possess both the form and function of hypnosis. As the next section discusses, the ritual of folk healing embodies many of the same components as the ritual of hypnosis. Individual sections then describe the hypothesis of the mechanism of action for hypnosis in the treatment of both burns and warts and the data supporting these hypotheses. Once the body's capability of healing in these two areas is demonstrated, the treatment of these two conditions by folk medicine, whether it functions by the precise mechanism of hypnosis or not, should be more believable.

Comparison of Hypnosis to Folk Healing

The Ritual

The ritualistic aspects of folk medicine and hypnosis are very similar and contribute to the effectiveness of the procedure. Especially striking are the parallels between healers such as those described in chapter three and professionally trained hypnotherapists. Both, for example, set the stage for the performance of their cure. In a clinical setting, the hypnotherapist will often have a special standardized induction which is paced according to the patient's responsitivity. Many hypnotherapists feel that the rate, tone, and quality of the voice are important in the induction of the trance and will vary their voices depending upon the stage of induction. Some inductions involve physically touching the patient, or holding an object in front of the patient to focus the person's gaze. Following a similar ritual, the folk healer generally uses a specific phrase or charm repeatedly. Burn healers, for example, may either chant the charm out loud or mumble it under their breath. They may wave their hands above the area, or blow gently upon it.

Confidence

Everyone who deals with the public knows that confidence makes any interaction go smoother, whether it's selling an appliance or discussing the efficacy of a drug. If the person making the pitch acts tentatively or insecurely the outcome is in jeopardy. The literature on placebo treatment clearly indicates that if a person has confidence in a procedure, the chances are greatly enhanced that the procedure will be effective. The corollary is also true that a person's doubts can decrease the efficacy of a proven effective medication. As one medical researcher has observed, "Any person will respond to a placebo given under conditions that galvanize that individual's belief" (Weil 209–10). Furthermore, "beliefs of practitioners about treatments are crucial determinants of therapeutic outcomes" (Weil 216).

Both the clinical hypnotherapist and the folk practitioner utilize confidence to facilitate their procedures. The hypnotherapist's confidence is generally developed by formal training in which the therapist has received close supervision initially in the procedure and then experienced successful outcomes. Obviously, the more experienced the practitioner and the greater the success, the more confidence he or she has in this procedure. When hypnotherapy is used by professionally trained practitioners, hypnosis is generally an adjunct to clinical practice. Hypnosis is, therefore, just one of a number of procedures that would be effective in achieving the desired results. For example, an anesthesiologist who uses hypnosis for anesthesia can also exercise a number of other clinical options to achieve similar results.

Warts

Because warts have been a human affliction through the centuries, it is not surprising that wart removal enjoys a rich history in the annals of folk medicine. Traditional folk approaches to the removal of warts can be found in much of southern literature, including Mark Twain's description of Huckleberry Finn's attempt to remove a wart by burying a cat at a crossroads at midnight. Some folk treatments of warts have involved other indirect approaches such as saying a charm over the wart or burying a poultice. Other methods, such as my father's wart being rubbed with a copper penny or a silk string being tied around a wart, have been somewhat more direct.

To understand how such folk cures work, we must know a little bit about warts in general and their natural course of growth and resolution once a person has acquired one. It is also important to have a general understanding of the basic immunology of warts in order to appreciate how hypnosis and folk procedures may cause them to disappear.

Pathology of Warts. Most warts are caused by the human papilloma virus (HPV), which is a member of a papovavirus group. Warts appear when a wart-producing virus invades the nucleus of skin cells called keratinocytes. Once the virus has invaded the skin, it increases the rate of division of the epidermal cells of the skin and causes the production of abnormal skin granules, which results in a thickening, folding, and increase in the horny layer of the skin. It used to be thought that all warts were caused by a single type of virus and that the site of infection determined the type of wart that would appear. Today, at least twelve different types of HPV have been found with more under study. Each type of wart has its own characteristic morphology and tends to have favorite areas it invades. For example, the common wart (HPV2, verruca vulgaris) is a smooth papule that usually occurs on the hand. It is also one of the two most common forms of warts (HPV2 and HPV6) that occur around the anus or on the genitalia of both males and females. The plantar wart (HPV1) is the rough elongated wart that is usually found on the sole of the foot. It is possible for a person to have several types of papilloma viruses producing different warts at the same time.

Spontaneous Remission. If left alone, most warts will spontaneously regress and disappear without treatment. Some authors have estimated that between 20 and 35 percent of all warts spontaneously regress in six months (Birkett). And one study, based on a survey involving one thousand children in an institution, found that 53 percent of the children who had warts lost them within one year and 63 percent within two years (Massing and Epstein).

Immunology of Warts. The mechanism of spontaneous wart remission is currently thought to be a result of the body's immunologic system combating the virus. This specific process in immunology is called cell mediated immunity. Once the body's immunologic system recognizes the virus as a foreign substance, a complex chain of events occurs in which specialized immunologic cells stimulate the rapid reproduction of B-cells and T-cells, which work to fight the current infections as well as to develop immunologic defense, which protects the body against future invasion by that same virus. Thus, when the body is exposed to the virus in the future, the B-cells and the T-cells kill or neutralize the virus before it can produce the rapid cell division and subsequent development of another wart.

The immune response is specific and will generally only protect against the specific type of virus against which it has previously mounted its immunologic attack. Some viruses so closely resemble each other that the body will mount an immunologic response against a new virus to which it has not been exposed because it so closely resembles a previous virus for which the immune system has developed protective antibodies. Thus, those people who have multiple warts as children or adolescents and appear to eventually "grow out of it" are thought to develop an immunologic response that not only clears the virus from the body but protects against future infection. As evidenced by the recurring nature of warts, the body's immunology protection may not be permanent, and a person may develop warts again after having been free of warts for some time. Some cell mediated immunity as well as the development of compliment fixing IgG antibodies appears to be the process whereby the body is able to rid itself of the virus and offer immunity against other infections (Birkett).

Medical Treatment of Warts. Birkett cites five basic ways that physicians currently treat warts: (1) Over-the-counter salicylic acid solutions; (2) Caustic topical treatment (acids); (3) Cryotherapy (freezing); (4) Electrocauterization (burning); and (5) Surgical removal. Each of these procedures has been found to be effective against warts, and the type of procedure used may depend upon the location of the wart. In addition, each procedure has its own risk, which is generally scarring of both the treated area and occasionally some of the surrounding normal tissue. The risk of scarring is an important consideration, given the evidence that so many warts resolve on their own without scarring.

Use of Hypnosis. For five decades articles have appeared in the medical and psychological journals describing the successful treatment of warts by the use of hypnosis. One of the earliest documented reports was by Bonjour, a physician who began treating warts by suggestion in 1888. Part of his procedure involved blindfolding the patient and touching the wart with his finger or a charm and giving the suggestion that the wart would disappear. Although details of his works are not available, he does report success.

As the use of hypnosis in the treatment of warts has continued, numerous practitioners have described their induction techniques and hypnotic suggestion in the treatment literature. Many practitioners use hypnotic suggestion to change the skin temperature at the site of the wart. Interestingly enough, success has been reported when either hand warmth or hand coolness has been used, as seen in Hartland, who used the hypnotic suggestion of warmth in the hands as opposed to Crasilneck and Hall, who used the sensation of coolness to remove the warts. Others have simply used the suggestion of the sensation of the skin tingling such as Surman, Gottlieb, and Hackett, who describe these suggestions as being successful in the treatment of a young girl with thirty-one warts.

In addition to publishing articles describing the use of hypnosis in removal of warts, various researchers have attempted to investigate the parameters of this phenomenon. One of the most obvious questions is whether or not hypnosis actually accounts for the removal of the warts, given the fact that there is spontaneous regression in the warts without intervention. Demonstrating that hypnosis, rather than the passage of time, is responsible for the removal of warts necessitates using control groups of subjects who have warts but are not undergoing hypnosis to see if they, too, experience the elimination of warts during this same period of time. A number of such studies (Barber; Sinclair-Geben and Chalmer) have been conducted using control groups not receiving treatment to control for the spontaneous regression of warts, and they have found that no warts disappeared in any of the entry control groups during the time that subjects receiving hypnosis were experiencing a disappearance of their warts.

Other researchers have attempted to demonstrate the specificity of hypnosis on warts by using a person as his or her own control group. In this case, a person who has warts on both sides of the body is given suggestions to remove warts on only one part of the body while no suggestions are given to eliminate warts on the opposite side of the body. Although one study has demonstrated the efficacy of this procedure, other researchers have reported that using hypnotic suggestion to remove warts on one side of the body produced this result on both sides. An explanation for the inability of hypnosis to treat a limited area of the body while leaving untreated another part of the body similarly infected has to do with the systemic nature of the immunologic system. For all the body except the brain, there is a general dissemination and equilibration of blood and its various components. Since the components of the immunologic system are carried through the bloodstream, all parts of the body are equally exposed to the immunologic production; therefore, changes in the immunologic system that would attack an invading virus on one part of the body would equally attack that virus found in other parts of the body.

Burns

All those who have rushed for the butter in the refrigerator or an aloe plant on the windowsill after burning themselves in the kitchen may be justifiably skeptical when hearing that folk healers can talk fire out of burns. When over-the-counter preparations and home remedies do little to shorten the persistent pain of even a small burn, the idea that both the pain and blistering caused by more severe burns can be lessened by having a chant spoken over them stretches the limits of credulity. Yet in chapter three Kirkland has given an eloquent description of the charms used by folk healers to talk fire out of burns, as well as providing brief case vignettes of successful treating of burn patients by folk healers who "talk fire out of burns."

That such healers continue to practice suggests that the burn patient receives some benefit from their intervention. Without some success the practitioner would quickly cease to function because no one would waste time on a procedure that did not bring relief from pain. Further attesting to the effectiveness of these folk healers is their relationship with some physicians in certain rural communities. In areas where fire is routinely talked out of burns, some physicians will admit patients to the hospital for the usual care of burn patients but will allow the folk practitioners full access to patients requesting their assistance.

My own experience with these practitioners is that they exist in larger numbers—especially in the South—than is generally recognized by the medical community. I can recall a number of years ago telling a patient that I would not be able to see him the following week because I would be out of town. When asked the nature of my absence, I mentioned that I was going to present a paper on the medical explanation of talking fire out of burns. The patient was a very pleasant gentleman in his mid-60s whom I had seen on a number of occasions and on whom I had obtained a rather complete psychosocial history. I was quite interested, as well as surprised, to learn that he talked fire out of burns. He proceeded to give me a number of case examples including one involving his own child. As a young man, the patient was shaving from a bowl of hot water at the foot of a shaving stand, when his toddler son accidentally fell into the water. My patient quickly picked up his crying son and invoked his charm to relieve the pain. In a matter of minutes his son stopped crying, cried no more from pains from the burn, and had no blistering or scarring from the event.

The relationship between hypnosis and burns has long been established by a very intriguing demonstration. Under a hypnotic trance, a subject can be touched with an object at room temperature and be told that the object is very hot. The area just touched by the cool object will begin to redden and will produce a blister with a precise outline of the object. This can be a very dramatic demonstration of hypnosis when viewed for the first time. In a similar way, a subject can be touched with a very hot object, but be told that the object is cool, and subsequently develop neither the redness nor blistering of the area that would be expected.

Given the demonstration that the human body can both develop a burn response to a cool object and block a blister response to a hot object, it is not surprising to learn that hypnosis has been used successfully by the medical community in the treatment of burned patients. Crasilneck and Hall are credited with describing the first demonstrated effectiveness of hypnotic procedures in the management of burn patients in modern medical literature. In this study the researchers reported relief from pain, an increase in appetite, and a reduction of psychological regression and negativism, which usually result from burn trauma.

One dramatic case that appears in the literature is from Dr. Dabney Ewin (1983), who describes the use of hypnosis with a patient of his who had slipped into a pot of molten aluminum. The patient's right leg went into molten aluminum at 900 Centigrade, an accident that would normally produce full thickness third degree burns and be very susceptible to infection. He was taken to the hospital where he was hypnotized within thirty minutes of his accident. He developed only a second degree burn, no antibiotics were used with the patient, and he developed no subsequent infection. He was discharged from the hospital on the nineteenth day and healed without scar tissue formation on the leg.

Today, there is a growing medical literature of single case and multiple case reports of hypnosis being used effectively with burned patients. One of the most important initial effects of hypnosis with a patient is in the area of pain control. Many practitioners use the hypnotic suggestion of the anesthesia. It is interesting that certain authors, such as Ewin, warn against using the word "normal," stating that when this was done in experimental subjects studies, some of those subjects did develop a "normal" burn. Through its general effect, hypnosis appears to reduce the burn depth and decrease the body's inflammatory reaction, thus reducing the amount of scarring, if any, that occurs after a burn.

Without the protective covering of the skin the fluids in our body would evaporate quickly and we would die. This is a very real danger facing patients suffering from significant burns over a large portion of their body, for exposed areas provide for rapid fluid loss by dehydration and oftentimes patients die due to complications of fluid management. Compounding the problem is the fact that burn patients often do not feel like eating or drinking and have a difficult time taking in the amount of fluid that is needed to keep ahead of the evaporation-dehydration process. Hypnotic suggestions have proved to be very effective in increasing the amount of fluid and food that the burned patient will take in. Therefore, in addition to the much needed pain relief that hypnosis can provide, it also has proven to facilitate other components of healing that have long-term benefits, including decrease in scarring, fluid loss, and electrolyte imbalance, thereby shortening the hospital stay.

Although hypnosis has been empirically shown to be effective in the treatment of burns, many researchers have been interested in the mechanism by which it produces its healing effect. The body's natural response to a burn is that of inflammation, which can consist of a series of symptoms, including burning pain, tenderness, swelling, fever, and blistering. Landmark work in this area was conducted by Chapman, Goodell, and Wolff, who demonstrated that during the first two hours after a burn injury, a bradykinin-like substance associated with inflammatory response is released, causing a progressive, pathologic worsening of the injury.

They, and others, have shown that "damaging inflammatory reaction can be blocked by early hypnosis, attenuating the ultimate depth and severity of a burn" (Ewin 1983, 5). By using hypnotic suggestion, doctors have been able to reduce the edema in the area of the burn caused by increased capillary permeability, thus reducing the damage done by plasma proteins and fluids from the blood vessels leaking into the inner-tissue areas. By blocking the bradykinins and histamine leaking into tissue space, hypnosis prevents the accelerating of the inflammatory response.

The mechanism by which hypnosis accomplishes these effects has not been demonstrated. Most practitioners use the hypnotic suggestion of coolness in the area of a burn to help reduce pain and swelling. Normally, coolness in the skin results from a process called vasoconstriction of the vessels, in which the diameter of the blood vessel becomes smaller, thus allowing less blood per unit of time to flow through it. The result is that the blood must take alternative routes from the vessels close to the skin's surface. As less warm blood flows beneath the surface of the skin, the temperature of the skin drops, thus producing the cool feeling. It is, therefore, possible that vasoconstriction of the blood vessels protects vascular integrity as well as reduces the amount of histamine and bradykinins that reach the area of injury. As indicated earlier, the practitioners of this technique suggest that the hypnotic suggestion must be given as early as possible and hopefully within minutes to hours of the burn. There is some indication that if hypnosis is not used during the first hours after a burn, it can still be useful, but in a different way. It is well known that an inadequate blood supply to a wound will result in a much delayed wound healing while also increasing the chance of infection. Moore and Kaplan describe the effective use of vasodilation by hypnosis in the healing of burn wounds when the hypnosis was begun one day after the burn occurred.

The patients used were those that had symmetrical or bilateral equivalent burns on some portion of their right and left sides, usually their hands. An hypnotic trance was induced and they were given suggestions to induce vasodilation on only one of the burn sides. Skin temperature was measured using an electrothermometer. The subject was able to serve as his or her own control group and thereby compare the differential healing effects of hypnosis. Four of the five patients demonstrated accelerated healing on the side which was treated with hypnotically induced vasodilation. The fifth patient elevated the temperature on both hands to the same extent, and it was felt that rapid healing occurred on both sides.

It is interesting to note that the authors felt that the fifth patient had consciously or subconsciously elected to increase the blood flow to both hands in order to obtain maximum healing.

The literature suggests that healing by hypnosis works by different mechanisms in different states of the burn. Initially, a sense of coolness and vasoconstriction reduces the inflammatory response, which reduces the amount of tissue damage. Later, vasodilation allows the rapid reestablishment of metabolic homeostasis to the area of burn. These findings are similar to the standard treatment in sports medicine in which the initial treatment for bruise or sprain is cold packs immediately after the injury and dry heat a day or two later.

In summary, hypnosis appears to effect the healing of burns by three separate measures. First, there is immediate relief to the patient by the reduction in pain. Second, hypnosis reduces the extension of the injury by reducing the initial inflammatory response. Later hypnosis promotes healing by increased blood flow, which stabilizes area metabolism and carries away waste products and damaged tissue. Thus the treatment of burns is an excellent example of hypnosis being used to help the body do something it is capable of doing, but that is not normally under conscious control. Each of these mechanisms occurs at its own pace, but induced at the appropriate time by hypnosis, their effects are significantly increased to the benefit of the patient.

It seems likely, therefore, that many practitioners of hypnosis have been able to use a hypnotic trance in treating burn patients without having any idea of the physiology of a burn. In spite of their ignorance, a hypnotic trance has been induced, suggestions of comfort, coolness, or recovery have been given, and very complex physiological changes have occurred, often without the slightest idea by the practitioner of what has occurred. Even today our knowledge of what actually happens to speed healing under hypnosis is very limited; yet, in spite of our not knowing the precise mechanism and all the processes which occur, such responses continue to occur when hypnosis is used.

I would suggest that when a folk healer reaches the bedside of a person severely burned a similar mechanism occurs. The healer may not have any awareness of the inflammatory response or the effect that the treatment procedure will have on the burn wound itself. Nonetheless, there is irrefutable evidence that many patients have benefited from such practitioners. With our scientific minds, we rightfully search for the mechanism that makes such a response possible. But the discovery of new information also means that our knowledge is incomplete. The concepts of vasoconstriction or vasodilation which are vitally important to the healing of any wound are necessarily very general concepts and have many smaller and more complex steps that are often unknown and extremely difficult to monitor from a research point of view.

There may also be other complex and unexpected processes involved that do not lend themselves to research. Some of the responses such as pain control could fall under the title that is generally thought of as "placebo" response. In the past a placebo was not thought to produce any real change in body metabolism or physiology. But when the placebo was given to someone it produced the desired effect, such as pain control or going to sleep. It was called a placebo because the substance was thought to have no properties of its own to produce the effect that occurred.

Recent studies have shown, however, that placebos work in some people by stimulating the body's own painkillers, called endorphins and encephlins, which can be as effective in controlling pain as opiates such as heroin or morphine. When taken normally, the placebo produces no increase in endorphins and encephlins, but when the suggestion of pain relief is given, the body releases these natural painkillers, producing a reduction of pain by chemicals that are true painkillers. Thus it appears that any placebos that would normally appear to effect no real change in the body can, in fact, produce very dramatic changes that have heretofore been unknown and unexpected. Research is underway to test whether or not hypnosis may also control pain by the release of the body's natural endorphins and encephlins.

Another exciting area that may relate to the effectiveness of hypnosis lies in the burgeoning area of psychoimmunology. It has been observed for eons that stress affects peoples' physical well-being, but it has only been within the last ten years that research has begun to allow us to explore precisely how this happens. Research has shown that stress, such as the death of a spouse, can directly influence the person's physical well-being by decreasing a specific class of immunoglobulins which serve to fight off various illnesses. People with this reduced level of immunoglobulins were shown to have an increased incidence of illness, thus providing the first link between stress and a mechanism that affected a person's health. These are the same components of the immune system which are involved in fighting viruses that cause warts and the inflammatory response that is stimulated after a burn. It is possible that hypnosis exerts its healing influence in part by a direct effect upon the immune system. In the case of burns, it may block an arm of the immune system that stimulates and intensifies the inflammatory response, thus reducing the resultant tissue damage produced by inflammation. Warts may receive an opposite effect in which blood flow is actually increased to the area of the wart, thus bringing an increase in the blood-borne immunoglobulins that fight viral infections. By an unknown process, hypnosis might help stimulate the production of the class of immunoglobulins that fight the virus.

The hypothesis for changes in blood flow and increase or decrease of the immune system may seem contradictory and thus not possible by the same process. However, reflecting on an earlier example of hypnosis will show how this is possible. Hypnosis has been shown to raise a blister from a cool object, a result that demonstrates the ability of this procedure to decrease the integrity of blood vessels, allowing fluids to increase their flow to areas not normally seen. Hypnosis has also been shown to decrease blistering caused by a hot object, thus demonstrating an opposite effect. Therefore, evidence exists showing both the increase and decrease of blood flow in different situations.

As with the procedures involving the effectiveness of placebos, psychoimmunology research techniques are new, expensive, and difficult to apply in the area of hypnosis research. My prediction is, however, that as our sophistication in research increases, we will find many more commonalities between placebo therapy, hypnosis, and folk healing, and very powerful changes in the body's normal corrective physiology will most likely be shown to be similar in all three areas. For example, I think the role of stimulating the body's own opiates will be shown to be a common explanation for pain relief in both hypnosis and folk healing. Even more complex induction of psychoimmunology will be shown to account for many powerful and direct treatment effects previously felt to be beyond conscious control.

References

Allington, H. V. "Review of the Psychotherapy of Warts." *Archives of Dermatology and Syphiology* 66 (1952): 316–26.

Barber, T. X. "Suggested ('Hypnotic') Behavior: The Trance Paradigm vs. an Alternative Paradigm." *Hypnosis: Research Developments and Perspectives.* Ed. E. Fromm and R. Shor. Chicago: Aldine, 1972.

Birkett, D. A. "Warts and Their Management." *The Practitioner* 226 (1982): 1,251–54.

Bonjour, J. "Influence of the Mind on the Skin." *British Journal of Dermatology* 41 (1929): 324–26.

Campo, M. S. "Warts and All." *Nature* 298 (1982): 605–6.

Chapman, L. F., H. Goodell, and H. G. Wolff. "Increased Inflammatory Reaction Induced by Central Nervous System Activity." *Transactions of the Association of American Physicians* 72 (1959): 84–110.

Crasilneck, H. P., and J. A. Hall. *Clinical Hypnosis: Principles and Application.* New York: Grune, 1975.

Crasilneck, H. P., J. A. Stirman, B. J. Wilson, et al. "Use of Hypnosis in the Management of Patients with Burns." *Journal of the American Medical Association* 158 (1955): 103–6.

Curtis, Helena. *The Viruses.* New York: National History Press, 1965.

Ewin, D. M. "Condyloma Acuminatum: Successful Treatment of Four Cases of Hypnosis." *American Journal of Clinical Hypnosis* 17.2 (1974): 73–78.

———. "Clinical Use of Hypnosis for Attenuation of Burn Depth." *Hypnosis at Its Bicentennial.* Ed. F. Frankel and H. Zamansky. New York: Plenum, 1978. 155–62.

———. "Emergency Room Hypnosis for the Burned Patient." *American Journal of Clinical Hypnosis* 26.1 (1983): 5–8.

Gravitz, M. A. "The Production of Warts by Suggestion as a Cultural Phenomenon." *American Journal of Clinical Hypnosis* 23.4 (1981): 281–83.

Hartland, J. "Hypnosis in Dermatology." *British Journal of Clinical Hypnosis* 1 (1970): 2–7.

Johnson, R. F., and T. X. Barber. "Hypnosis, Suggestions, and Warts: An Experimental Investigation Implicating the Importance of 'Believed-in Efficacy.'" *American Journal of Clinical Hypnosis* 20.3 (1978): 165–74.

Fenton, M. J. "Hypnosis and Dermatology." *Hypnosis and Behavioral Medicine* (1965): 91–95.

Margolis, C. G., B. B. Domangue, D. Ehleben, and L. Shrier. "Hypnosis in the Early Treatment of Burns: A Pilot Study." *American Journal of Clinical Hypnosis* 26.1 (1983): 9–15.

Massing, A. M., and W. L. Epstein. "Natural History of Warts." *Archives of Dermatology* 87 (1963): 306–10.

Moore, L. E., and J. Z. Kaplan. "Hypnotically Accelerated Burn Wound Healing." *American Journal of Clinical Hypnosis* 26.1 (1983): 16–19.

Schafer, D. W. "Hypnosis Use on a Burn Unit." *The International Journal of Clinical and Experimental Hypnosis* 23.1 (1974): 1–14.

Sheehan, D. V. "Influence of Psychosocial Factors on Wart Remission." *American Journal of Clinical Hypnosis* 20.1 (1978): 160–64.

Sinclair-Geben, A. H., and D. Chalmer. "Treatment of Warts by Hypnosis." *Lancet* 2 (1959): 480–82.

Surman, O. S., S. K. Gottlieb, and T. P. Hackett. "Hypnotic Treatment of a Child with Warts." *American Journal of Clinical Hypnosis* 15 (1972): 12–14.

Wakeman, R. J., and J. Z. Kaplan. "An Experimental Study of Hypnosis in Painful Burns." *American Journal of Clinical Hypnosis* 21.1 (1978): 3–12.

Weil, A. *Health and Healing: Understanding Conventional and Alternative Medicine.* Boston: Houghton Mifflin, 1983.

5. Doctors and Root Doctors: Patients Who Use Both

Holly F. Mathews

In this essay I will describe a traditional ethnomedical system known as "root medicine" or "rootwork" which has been well documented primarily among black Americans, but which also influences health behaviors among white and Native Americans in the rural South and in the ghetto areas of most of the larger metropolitan areas in the North and Midwest (see Mathews 886 for more information on the geographic distribution of these beliefs). My goal is to demonstrate how the often seemingly bizarre beliefs and practices espoused by adherents of the system make sense within the traditional historical and cultural context of the region. Because these beliefs and practices continue to satisfy a number of the group's psychological and physical health needs which are not met by available modern care, they influence significantly the ways in which adherents participate in encounters with and respond to treatments received from mainstream physicians. Ultimately, such an analysis must consider the issue of effectiveness by asking how satisfactory the ethnomedical system is in meeting the health needs of the people it serves (cf., Foster and Anderson 51). I will attempt to answer this question from the "emic" point of view, that is, from the point of view of the adherents themselves. In chapter six Peter Lichstein will examine the rootwork system from the clinician's perspective.

My analysis draws upon fieldwork on rootwork conducted between 1978 and 1982 in three rural communities and in clinical settings in the central Piedmont region of North Carolina, and between 1985 and 1991 in ten rural counties and associated clinical settings in the coastal plain of eastern North Carolina.[1] During this period I have conducted in-depth interviews and have observed patient sessions with nine practicing root doctors and five herbalists. In addition, I have talked with lay midwives, women and men who specialize in preparing home remedies, and with ministers and religious healers of various types along with the people who seek them out for help in the treatment of illness in these communities. My analysis also draws upon a set of interviews done with a sample of rural elders in eastern North Carolina about their use of alternative and mainstream medical care.

In the first half of this essay I present a composite description of the rootwork system distilled from all of these sources. I acknowledge that it is rare for any single individual to be able to articulate the complete model of illness and treatment presented here. While some individuals, most notably the healers, have fairly extensive knowledge of rootwork beliefs and practices, others, particularly occasional users of the system, do not. They may remember isolated beliefs and have only limited knowledge of home or herbal remedies, yet they may still call upon traditional explanatory models for understanding and traditional healers for assistance when they think that modern medicine has failed them.

As Hufford notes in chapter one, composite descriptions, no matter how useful, are still intellectual devices. While they help present a picture of the relations that obtain between sometimes seemingly disconnected beliefs and practices, they do not necessarily tell us anything about what individuals think and do. Moreover, no individual, as Hufford writes, "ever *completely* replicates a single tradition. There are always idiosyncracies and there are usually signs of influence from other traditions" (24). Consequently, it is equally important that the investigator determine how the integrated system of knowledge given in the composite picture is actually drawn upon by individuals in constructing explanations for illness and in making decisions about appropriate treatments. In the second half of this essay I use case studies to illustrate the ways in which traditional beliefs influence individual patient encounters with and expectations of mainstream medical personnel.

History and Description of the Rootwork System

The traditional medicine of black Americans is known generally as "rootwork" or "root medicine" because plant roots are an important component of the magical spells that are used to cause illnesses and of the remedies used to cure them (Mathews 885). Equally characteristic, however, is a belief in the natural causation of illness and the possibility of cure with herbs and other natural medicines. The system is based on a view of life as a union of body, mind, and soul, and a definition of health as the blending of physical, social, and emotional well-being. Its followers, like a majority of the world's peoples, are now and historically have been medically pluralistic (compare Wallis and Morley). Treatment is sought from a variety of practitioners, none of whom is thought to have a monopoly over the ability to cure.

The origins of black traditional medicine can be traced to slave culture in the antebellum South (see Jordan; Levine; Snow 1983; Savitt). Slaves, brought to the United States from a variety of tribal groups in Africa, faced starvation and disease with the only techniques they had available—magical and herbal cures from their homelands. The traditional African medicine man, known as the conjurer, juju man, sorcerer, or witchdoctor, was a general practitioner who cured not only with herbs, but who also acted as an intermediary with various divinities and as a manipulator of magical forces (Jackson). Over time, as slaves from different tribal groups shared cures among themselves; borrowed additional herbal lore and curative practices from Native Americans; and adopted the colonial European use of purgatives, bleedings, and preventive measures based on classical humoral pathology (Pockrein; Savitt); a new, amalgamated ethomedical system evolved. Yet the form of the evolving medical system varied along with the specific locality of the slave group.

In the Caribbean, traditional African religious beliefs blended well with the structurally similar cosmology of Catholicism as practiced by the European planters. This created a belief system known as voodoo, where illness and misfortune involved primarily religious and magical causes and cures (see Tinling; Jordan). Voodoo was transplanted subsequently to the area around New Orleans, where the slave trade and movement of planters from the Caribbean were most active (Tallant). In other areas of the Southeast, however, the religious role of the conjurer came to a rapid end with the conversion of slaves to Protestant forms of Christianity some 200 years after settlement in the New World (McCall). Magic was decried by Protestant denominations as the work of the Devil, and religious healing was undertaken exclusively by church-sanctioned personnel, including ministers and lay spiritual leaders. The traditional conjurer, however, continued to serve an important role in slave culture, treating illness with herbal remedies and practicing magic (Levine; McCall; Snow 1983). Magic is the belief that supernatural forces can be controlled and manipulated by humans to gain advantage over others. It is found in most traditional cultures and tends to prevail, as the anthropologist Malinowski observed, under situations of uncertainty when people perceive an insufficient knowledge or lack of control over events in their world.

Certainly slave society exhibited these conditions. Removed from their traditional lands and ways of life, slaves faced not only physical hardships but also psychological alienation (Levine). Kept at the bottom of a rigid social caste system, slave lives were characterized by a sense of uncertainty, a feeling of hopelessness, and a fear of the future. For them, the practice of magic to both cause and cure misfortune served several practical and perhaps valuable functions. First, a belief in magic enabled slaves to regain some feeling of control over a hopeless situation and in the process acted to preserve health and sanity. Second, magic offered slaves a source of power and knowledge not possessed by their white masters. As such it provided a unifying identity for slaves from diverse cultural backgrounds. It is not surprising, therefore, that magic helped give many slaves the courage to persevere and even to rebel against their oppressors. Finally, magical beliefs functioned as a source of internal social control in slave communities lacking established methods of dispute settlement. The threat of retaliation by magic was often enough to encourage slaves to abide by social norms. Magic thereby helped to create and preserve some form of community organization for slaves living in unstable and unpredictable situations.

After the Civil War, the customs and policies of the controlling class of southern whites continued to deny most rural blacks access to mainstream health care and thus fostered their continued reliance on this ethnomedical system, perpetuating its survival long after such ethnomedical practices had become moribund in other groups (compare Jackson).

Today the key practitioners in the system are known as "root doctors" or "conjurers" because of their role in casting spells known as "hexes" or "roots" and in curing people afflicted by magically induced illness. The belief in root magic, however, is but one small part of the more comprehensive ethnomedical tradition which combines a belief in the magical causation of illness with a naturalistic disease etiology and an acceptance of Protestant Christian theology (see also Snow 1983; Hill). According to the logic of this system, the individual lives in a hostile world where the forces of God are pitted against the forces of the Devil in a daily struggle for control. Illness and misfortune are likely to result whenever the individual fails to maintain a balance between these competing forces,

Table 5.1 Treatment Options for Different Categories of Disease

	Natural Cause	Unnatural Cause
Body Problems	*natural cure:* home remedies, herbalist, pharmacist, chiropractor, physician	*magical cure:* root doctor
Mind Problems	*spiritual cure:* prayer, minister, faith healer, spiritualist	*magical cure:* root doctor

whether natural or magical. The traditional system makes a distinction between illnesses of the mind and of the body and between illnesses having natural as opposed to unnatural causes. These distinctions have implications for treatment choice (see table 5.1). Natural illnesses occur when individuals fail to maintain harmony in the physical or spiritual world. Unnatural illnesses, by contrast, are believed to stem directly from the evil acts of others who use magic for their own gain (see figure 5.1).

Natural Illnesses

Natural illnesses are those which result from a violation of the balance or harmony believed to be present in the physical world. According to this belief system, the forces of nature and the human body exist in a state of harmony in God's world. It is the responsibility of the individual to monitor bodily processes, take care of himself, and make sure that the harmonic balance of the body is not disturbed. Moderation becomes the guide for daily living because excesses like overeating, staying out late, or going out into the cold without adequate clothing can potentially upset bodily balance and lead to illness (see also Hill and Mathews; Hill; Snow 1983).

The classification of natural illnesses is based on a well-organized system of belief in which the key to health is maintaining a proper balance and flavor in the blood. Blood that is out of balance may not only be too sweet or bitter, but it may also be too high or low, too thick or thin, or too dirty (see also, Moerman; Hill and Mathews; Mathews; and Snow 1974, 1977, 1983). The concepts of pressure and flavor are linked in this system such that blood that is too high is often thought to be too sweet while blood that is too low is often thought to be too bitter. Specifically, high and low blood are folk illness categories that refer to the amount and location of blood in the body. Each type of imbalance is believed to lead to a different set of illnesses grouped under the controlling organs of the

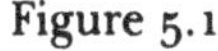

Figure 5.1

Taxonomy of Folk Illnesses

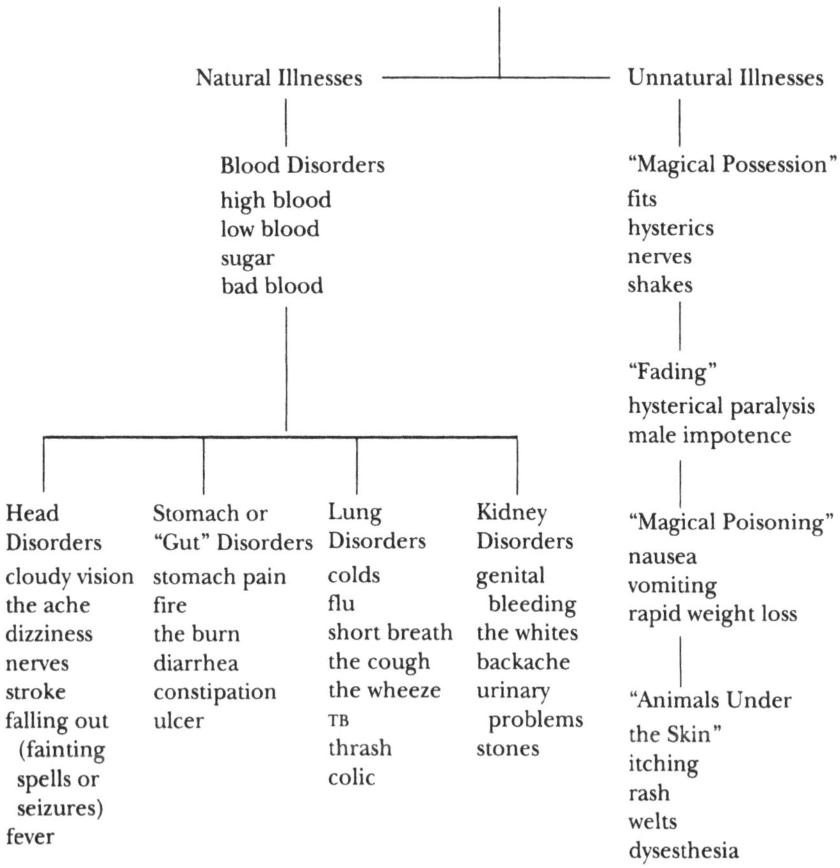

- Natural Illnesses
  - Blood Disorders: high blood, low blood, sugar, bad blood
    - Head Disorders: cloudy vision, the ache, dizziness, nerves, stroke, falling out (fainting spells or seizures), fever
    - Stomach or "Gut" Disorders: stomach pain, fire, the burn, diarrhea, constipation, ulcer
    - Lung Disorders: colds, flu, short breath, the cough, the wheeze, TB, thrash, colic
    - Kidney Disorders: genital bleeding, the whites, backache, urinary problems, stones
- Unnatural Illnesses
  - "Magical Possession": fits, hysterics, nerves, shakes
  - "Fading": hysterical paralysis, male impotence
  - "Magical Poisoning": nausea, vomiting, rapid weight loss
  - "Animals Under the Skin": itching, rash, welts, dysesthesia

body: the head, the lungs, the stomach or "gut," and the kidney (see figure 5.1). Each illness consists of a set of "signs" or associated symptoms. These symptoms, however, are not exclusive to particular illnesses; rather, the same sets of symptoms may be classified differently depending upon the perceived cause of the problem (Mathews 887).

Natural illnesses can be subdivided into those of the body and those of the mind (Mathews 887–88). Natural body problems result from this failure of the individual to maintain bodily harmony and are considered amenable to treatment with natural remedies. Most adherents of the rootwork system practice prevention on a regular basis. They employ a wide variety of tonics, herbal treatments, and dietary regulations to try and maintain balance. When illness does result, the first recourse for natural, body problems is the use of home remedies that incorporate these traditional herbal components as well as over-the-counter medications. If the condition persists or increases in severity, then the individual may seek out a specialist in herbal treatments, either a knowledgeable friend or practicing herbalist, for additional remedies. Generally, the people surveyed in my research agree that home and herbal remedies work effectively to cure most minor, natural ailments. While they think a physician's medicines are "stronger and more powerful" than most herbs, they also see these medicines as being more dangerous and less healthy than "natural, plant remedies."

It is apparent from my own research, however, that the knowledge of herbal medicine is unevenly distributed in the local population. In any given rural community, there may be one, or at most two, practicing herbalists. Most of these traditional herbalists have many years of experience in collecting and preparing plants, know the properties of many different varieties and species, and have observed over time the empirical effects of their remedies on different illnesses. In addition, most report having received a special calling from God to the role—a calling made apparent in unusual signs at birth and special abilities manifested in youth. All report a desire to do the Lord's work and to serve others without worry about monetary compensation.

Mrs. Emma Dupree, for example, is a ninety-four-year-old herbalist living in the town of Fountain, North Carolina. Her birth on July 4 was marked by special signs. As she says, "When I was born, I was the seventh one, the seventh sister, and they say the seventh one will be over-endowed in everything." At the time of her birth, the family reported a glow that stayed around the house until 10 A.M. As Mrs. Dupree interpreted: "[My mother] says that's why I was so different. I was a different child. People talked and I listened and my heart was big enough to hold all that. I talked different . . . was strong in my talking . . . I was just born to that" (quoted in Baldwin 50). As she grew older, Mrs. Dupree's calling became more apparent. She spent a lot of time in the woods observing nature and was always interested in the healing power of plants. She remembers, "The woods gal, that's what they called me. They'd say, here comes that little medicine thing" (Baldwin 50). She would help anyone who asked, often making long trips on foot to visit the sick and bring herbal cures to those in need. As she says, "I always did it. There wasn't nobody sick nowhere around me, around Falkland, white or colored, but that I wouldn't be there" (Baldwin 50). Mrs. Dupree also worked for a time for a local white doctor and learned from him as well: "I've learned a lot though from the doctor, helping him out with his medicine, and keeping it all straight on the shelf and making his herbs, and then the doctor lady, I'd go with her in the night to get herbs. And she'd take pains and show me what type grew where and what the roots looked like. That was all the help I had" (Dupree 4). Her real ability to heal and all of her successes, however, she attributes to Jesus. As she explains it: "Jesus. And I don't talk about it unless I am talking to Him about it . . . the powerhouse, Jesus, for everything we made, He made it. He put life and power in everything. He created the earth, the air, the wind, and everything. All power belongs to him" (*Little Medicine Thing*). Traditional herbalism, however, is a skill that appears to be dying out as the existing practitioners grow old. All of the herbalists I interviewed reported difficulty in finding young people who were interested in herbs or willing to learn more about healing. Mrs. Dupree laments the changing times as she foresees the end of her career:

> But in these places it [herbs] don't grow like it did . . . down around Falkland down by the river. The people and the children growing up then lived off of them. 'Twas very scientific. And they don't get none of that now, and it makes them different. Their blood is not fed with it—with stuff like back when I was growing up. And after I was grown, I've still used this [herbs] and the old people did too. But just like everything else, it changes. I said if my mamma could come back and see all this stuff now, I expect she'd dig a hole and run right back in the ground. And see all that is happening in this life now is going on from the way back and the way back is still the best. Ain't it true? And it [herbs] makes me very strong and prissy and great and thanking to God. That's like He made it, and that's the way I am. [*Little Medicine Thing*].

In addition to the practicing herbalists, most older adults in the communities surveyed grew two or three herbs in their yards, recognized a few more that grew in the wild, and knew how to make a limited number of standard remedies which they often supplied to younger family members and friends. Among the younger generation of adults aged forty and less, knowledge of plant species and the preparation of remedies was almost nonexistent, although many of these individuals still thought that herbal remedies, of the type their mothers had made, were better than medicines. On occasion, those with limited knowledge suffered severe side effects from using poisonous plants or incorrectly prepared remedies (see Jaeckle and Freemon for a case example). As Croom points out in chapter eight, herbal remedies can have severe side effects and are sometimes toxic. Traditional herbalists know a great deal about both the properties of plants in the local region and about the proper ways to prepare them. As this knowledge is lost, the likelihood of mistakes increases.

Physicians also play a role in the treatment of natural illnesses. The choice process among the alternative therapies is a logical one. At the time of illness onset, if the condition is judged to be acute or particularly severe, a physician is chosen for treatment. Frequently, serious conditions are said to include accidents or severe infections. Alternatively, if an illness fails to respond to home remedies or herbal treatments, then the individual may seek the help of a physician. In either case, the individual approaches the medical encounter with very specific expectations of the physician which, if not shared by him, can lead to serious problems of miscommunication. Case examples of such miscommunication will be presented in the final section of this essay.

A natural illness that fails to respond to the usual treatments may eventually be reclassified on the basis of cause as a natural, mind problem sent as a punishment by God for a transgression or sin (see Mathews 888–89; Hill; and Snow 1983). In such a situation, the curing of the physical symptoms of the illness will not eliminate the problem because the ultimate cause of the condition (the sin) has not been resolved. Individuals who fail to deal with the spiritual aspects of the condition are believed to continue to suffer recurring physical symptoms. To cure a spiritual problem, an individual must seek the assistance of a minister, faith healer, or spiritual congregation to intercede with God and effect a cure. These religious practitioners mediate the confession of the sin by the offender and assist him or her in accepting forgiveness.

The case of Mrs. Jones, a fifty-year-old black female resident of a small coastal community in North Carolina, illustrates the course of treatment likely to be pursued for a natural illness as its cause is reconceptualized over time. I first met Mrs. Jones when I was interviewing her neighbor about herbal remedies. The neighbor told me that Mrs. Jones had been sick for quite a while with a persistent skin rash, headaches, and a general "logey" or fatigued feeling. Mrs. Jones told me that her problems had begun rather suddenly. She awoke one morning to find her arms and hands covered with an itchy rash. She thought at first that it was poison ivy since she had been working in the yard the day before. She used calamine lotion on the rash and took aspirin for her headache which she attributed to "overdoing it the day before." But her rash showed no signs of diminishing that week and so she asked her neighbor for help. The neighbor gave her an herbal poultice to place on the rash and a tonic to drink to "build up her blood to fight the infection." Mrs. Jones dutifully took the preparation but to no avail. By the next week, the rash had spread to her legs and stomach. She still felt tired and achy and was becoming worried. When her daughter came to visit, she told her about the worsening condition. In the process of the discussion, her daughter made the following statement: "You know, you wasn't talkin' about this sickness 'til that day you had that match with Miss Mary at the church. Are you sure all that arguin' didn't upset you? Maybe you is jus' sick over all that business in the church." More discussion followed. Mrs. Jones told the neighbor about the incident that Sunday. She reported that after church as the congregation went out back to eat a covered dish lunch, she heard Miss Mary and the other members of the Pastor's Committee criticizing her for not bringing any food to the lunch. Mrs. Jones said that she marched right up to them and told them that she hadn't brought any food because she didn't have any to bring, and that it was a very un-Christian thing for them to criticize others. Well, the pastor overheard and scolded them all for quarreling on a Sunday. Mrs. Jones admitted that this incident had been bothering her all week. She had skipped church the Sunday after and said she was afraid to go back because she, "jus' couldn't face them ladies and the pastor." At this point, her daughter suggested that she go to see the pastor privately at his office and tell him about what happened that day and apologize. "Why should I be the one to apologize?" exclaimed Mrs. Jones, "I didn't start the whole thing." Her daughter answered: "Look, Mother, if you go first then you will seem bigger than these other ladies, and Pastor Peele will know that you are a good, Christian person and he won't be thinkin' the worst of you. Those other ladies are jus' small minded people. You are gettin' sick because of them. You go with the Lord on your side. Go on over. I'll go with you."

Mrs. Jones did indeed go to see the pastor that week, and when I saw her a few days later, all signs of her illness had disappeared. She had this to say:

> I guess I just kinda fooled myself. It was that upset makin' me sick. But I just couldn't do nothing to get out of it 'til Mavis told me to go see the pastor. And you know, he was jus' tickled I came 'cause he thought I was gonna leave the church and he said that he didn't want

> to lose me. And he told me that the Lord fed the crowds with only a loaf and a few fish and so our church could too, and that people who made on about others and worried others so about food were not being the kind of Christians they should be. So it made me feel a powerful lot better, you see, 'cause I knowed I had done the right thing goin' to him directly. And now I feel right with the Lord again and happy to sing his praises.

When I asked about her physical symptoms, she reported that the rash had disappeared and that she felt fine now because, "I cleared it with the Lord."

This case shows how an illness was first judged to be a natural, body problem and treated with over-the-counter and herbal remedies. When these failed to work, however, a discussion occurred in which the participants renegotiated the causal attribution determining that the physical symptoms had resulted instead from a spiritual problem. Once Mrs. Jones spoke with the minister, admitted her role in the incident at the church, and received his pardon, she was fine again. Her role as a church member and a good Christian, so vital to her personal identity, was restored (see chapter seven for a more extended discussion of the importance of identity conflicts in the onset of spiritual heart trouble among Pentecostals).

Unnatural Illnesses

Unnatural illnesses are those whose cause is located outside of the world of nature and natural causes (see figure 5.1). Unnatural problems can be subdivided into two groups: unnatural mind problems which result from the inability of the individual to cope with the stresses of everyday life, and unnatural body problems which result from the deliberate, evil acts of others or magic (see Mathews 889; Snow 1983, 826–27).

Unnatural mind problems are mental illnesses believed to occur when individuals magnify everyday problems to such proportions that they can no longer cope and simply "freak out" or "go crazy." Unnatural body problems are produced by spells, known as "roots" or "hexes,"[2] commissioned from a root doctor by a person who seeks to deliberately harm or gain control over another. For both types of problems, root doctors are the practitioner of choice (see also Hall and Bourne; Gums and Carson; Snow 1978).

The philosophical basis of the belief in the magical components of rootwork rests on the notion that some people are just born evil. These evil individuals seek to deliberately harm others. They are aided in this quest by the Devil, who has recruited them to work for him to spread evil in the world and thereby fight against God. The victims of rootwork are often those individuals who have lost God's protection because of sins committed in the past. When God's protection is suspended, these individuals are thought to be particularly susceptible to magical attacks. Treatment involves finding a root doctor who can reverse the spell or remove the hex.

The belief in the power of magic to achieve evil ends or to gain control over another person or uncertain life conditions is widespread among the adherents of the rootwork system. By definition, the illnesses suffered by the victims of magic are considered to be unnatural and hence are not considered amenable to ordinary treatments. Yet, as the medical literature demonstrates, many individuals who suspect that they are the victims of rootwork do end up in the medical system (compare Campinha-Bacote; Cappannari et al.; Freemon and Drake; Golden; Hillard and Rockwell; Kimball; McCall; Maduro; Saphir et al.; Wintrob; and Lichstein's essay, chapter six). How does this happen? The answer to this question is embedded in another, very important question: how can a person tell if he is indeed suffering from an unnatural illness?

Unnatural body problems are suspected if an individual suffers from certain physical symptoms associated traditionally with magical attacks (see Mathews 889). These focal symptoms of rootwork include the sensation of burning pain felt first in the extremities and then spreading all over the body. The pain is often accompanied by itching and the presence of a rash and is believed to be produced by the presence of animals under the skin, variously reported to include snakes, lizards, spiders, toads, and frogs. The spell itself is said to consist of a powder made from the eggs of one of these animals which is subsequently placed in the food of the intended victim. After the powder is eaten, the animals grow under the victim's skin, causing physical discomfort.

Other focal symptoms that signal rootwork include gastrointestinal complaints that are particularly severe or prolonged. For example, unexplained vomiting and nausea are believed to occur with magical poisoning. Similarly, rootwork is suspected in cases of hysterical paralysis known as "fading," which begins with a numbness in the legs and back that spreads all over the body until the victim is unable to walk. "Fading" is associated with impotence in men, and the victim's general lack of awareness of the world around him (similar to the zombie syndrome in voodoo). Finally, any kind of extremely strange or unusual behavior including having hallucinations, hearing voices, or doing abnormal things like running around without clothes on, may be attributed to rootwork.

The presence of any of these focal symptoms can be interpreted as a sure sign that someone has "put a root on" an individual. Alternatively, the individual may suspect that an illness is the result of rootwork if the root or spell itself is found. One man I interviewed, for example, found a small bottle containing the remains of a charred plant root buried in his backyard. He had not been sick before finding it, but immediately thereafter he developed the symptoms of "fading" and sought out a root doctor for help in removing the spell. Spells come in a variety of forms including roots in bottles; dolls or mud images that display a likeness to the intended victim (a form of sympathetic magic); red flannel bags containing something once in association with the victim like nail or hair clippings or pieces of clothing (a form of contagious magic); the bones of different animals; and even unusually colored stones. Often the residue of a spell, like the remains of grave dust sprinkled around a yard or over a door sill, may be found by the intended victim. Once the spell is found, a certain attribution of rootwork follows.

The actual evidence of a spell, however, is not necessary to suspect the perpetration of rootwork. It may be enough for the individual to simply suspect that someone is out to "get" him or to be told that someone "might mean to do him harm." Similarly, a person with a guilty conscience over an offense committed may eventually come to suspect that his victim has sought retribution by working a spell. In each of these cases the power of suggestion, either spread by the perpetrator of the spell through gossip or self-induced by the victim's own guilt, acts to bring on the individual's illness. I am frequently asked how often rootwork victims actually find spells and how often they suffer from suggestion. My data reveal that informants report actually finding spells in about 25 percent of the illness cases documented. In the rest they either spontaneously experienced a focal symptom, were told they had been hexed, or had a reason to suspect that someone was out to harm them. In the latter instance it is difficult to determine if the power of suggestion brought on a psychosomatic illness or if a coincident illness was interpreted by the victim to be the result of rootwork.

One final and very important way of determining that you are suffering from a root problem is to seek routine treatments or the help of a physician for an illness without experiencing any improvement in the original condition. As one of my informants put it: "Well, I'll tell you what. Now when a person goes to usin' this root stuff, the doctors can't do it no good. Ain't nothin' the doctor can do for you. The more you go to the doctor, the worse you gonna get 'cause the doctor'll tell you quick, 'You got somethin' I can't do nothin' with.' So you got to find out what's wrong yourself."

My informants believe that a person can suffer from rootwork without knowing it because evildoers are often able to disguise their evil from the victim. Thus, the afflicted individual will think he has a normal illness, take regular home remedies or see a doctor, and not suspect that something is wrong until he fails to get relief. Alternatively, they note that many people reject a belief in rootwork because it is seen to be a backward and superstitious or even evil custom and refuse to consider it as a possible cause of illness except as a last resort. Only when nothing else works will they consider rootwork as a possible cause.

Obviously, the considerations that go into determining the cause of illness and appropriate treatments are complex in the case of rootwork and may involve several episodes of reinterpretation. The following case illustrates these complexities. Veronica Stancil, a thirty-three-year-old black female, told me in some detail about a peculiar illness she had suffered the year before. Veronica lived at home with her mother and her young daughter, born out of wedlock. Veronica's mother had worked as a hotel maid in a local establishment until her ill health from diabetes and high blood pressure forced her to quit. She managed to work occasionally as a day maid, but the family's survival depended on the AFDC payment Veronica received and on small contributions from her child's father and his family. Prior to the onset of her illness, Veronica had begun working part-time for a middle-class, black family taking care of an elderly parent in the home while they worked. Veronica did not report her wages to the county welfare office and so was able to continue to receive public assistance as well. Between the money contributed by her child's father, her mother's occasional wages, public assistance, and the new job, her family was able to make ends meet for the first time in a long while. Veronica reported that she had been trying to put some money aside so that she could buy clothes and supplies for her daughter when she entered school. Everything was going well for the family until about two months after her job started. Veronica was able to pinpoint the onset of her illness to payday in the first week of the third month of her job. She described it this way:

> I was so happy 'bout gettin' paid that week 'cause I had found a couple of real pretty dresses at the aid shop that fit Jeannell [her daughter]. And I wanted to get them for her to wear to the party at the preschool that next day. And then when I got to work, they couldn't pay me 'cause they had to buy Mama Annie her medicines. So they said could they pay me double the next week. And so what could I say, them bein' so good to me an all. So I said ok, but then I worried all day 'bout them dresses. And so I thought I would jus' go by and see Jim [her daughter's father] after work and see if he or his mama would spot me for the dresses. Well, as soon as I got there, I saw him on the corner and he was talkin' to a girl I heard was goin' with him, and I jus' went on by 'cause I didn't want to make no trouble for him, you know. He's been good to me and all. So I went on by his house to see his mama. And he came after me and asked where I was goin' and I told him what I needed. And how Jeannell was goin' to be in a program at school and I wanted that dress. And he was fine. He said he didn't have nothin' right then but he was expectin' some money that evening and he'd bring some by the house tomorrow. So I said ok and went on in to see his mama. Well, I noticed how that girl of his was watchin' me the whole time but I didn't pay no attention to it. But the next day, I started feelin' so bad and sick, it was terrible. And when Jim came with the money, he knocked on the door, and I couldn't even talk with him I got so sick. I ran to the bathroom and threw up all over the place. So I never did see him. He left the money with my aunt. And I jus' kept gettin' sicker.

Veronica said that she thought she had a bug of some kind that wouldn't last long. So she went out and got the dresses but kept feeling worse. By Monday, she was very sick but still went to work. After work, she came home and collapsed. Her mother got very worried and made her drink some tea to ease the stomach. But she still wasn't better and so she went to the doctor the next day after work. He told her it was a flu bug and that she should rest, drink water, and take some pills he gave her. She did and began to feel well enough to keep working. But then, she said, she was leaving work one afternoon about a week later and got on the bus. She looked back and saw Jim there with his girl and right away began to feel sick. As Veronica put it, "I could hardly get off and to my house without falling out. As it was, I began to vomit again." When she told her mother and aunt of the incident, they began to suggest to her that her illness was being caused by someone else. As her mother said:

> Think back. Who was there when you first felt bad? Jim and his girl who kept staring at you. Then you was doin' better until you saw them again. It don't sound right to me. If this was some ordinary thing you'd be back to your feet by now. No, somethin' strange is goin' on here. I think that girl's got it in for you. She's jealous 'cause Jim still makes over you and the baby and gives you money. She wants him to herself. You know how these women can be over a man. You got to be careful.

Veronica began to think there could be something to her mother's idea and went to talk with Jim's mother about it. Jim's mother confirmed the interpretation saying that she had never liked the other girl because she, "jus' wasn't from good people." She advised Veronica to seek the help of a rootworker to find out what was wrong.

Veronica did visit a rootworker who told her that she had been bewitched by the girl. He told her the girl had had something put in her food that would make her sick every time she tried to see or talk to Jim. That way she hoped to keep Jim and her apart. He gave Veronica what she described as a potion to counteract the poison and a bag of powder to sprinkle in her shoes to keep away any other evil the girl might work. Veronica reported that she immediately recovered from her sickness and went and told Jim's mother the whole story. Jim's mother then decided to tell Jim and vowed that she "would do what I have to" to protect her son from the girl's evil ways.

This case illustrates the rootwork attribution process in some detail. Veronica began by assuming she had an ordinary, natural illness. She did nothing at first, waiting for it to go away. She next took home remedies and eventually saw a physician when the condition persisted. Although she found some relief from the symptoms, these recurred in a significant incident when she met her former boyfriend and his new woman on the bus. This episode of recurrence led to a discussion among Veronica's relatives as to the nature of her problem. A review of the social situation and events preceding her sickness led them to hypothesize that the illness was not, in fact, normal but rather was the result of evil intentions on the part of the other woman. This hypothesis was tested in conversations with Jim's mother who provided confirming support and was finally corroborated by the root doctor who then began to help Veronica with the situation. So although Veronica never found evidence of a spell, she did experience a focal symptom, gastrointestinal distress; she did try normal remedies without success; and she did have a reason to suspect someone was out to get her thanks to the suggestions of her family. In her eyes the rootwork attribution was the correct one since her illness was cured after the visit to the root doctor. The case also had the added effect of working to turn both Jim and his mother, important resource providers for Veronica's family, against the girlfriend, a potential drain on those resources. And Veronica's level of interpersonal stress, which she labeled at the time as "lettin' things get next to me," decreased significantly once the girlfriend ceased to be a threat. As to the "real" nature of Veronica's illness, we could assume it was psychosomatically induced or it may have been a coincidental trigger that provoked a resolution to a socially stressful situation. Either way, the symptoms she experienced were real to her and to her physician. Whether his medicines, the home remedies, the release of stress, the magic of the root doctor, or simply the passage of time cured her will never be known. The important point is that for Veronica, traditional medicine worked to solve both her physical and interpersonal problems.

It is the persistence of this magical component in the present-day rootwork system that most puzzles mainstream health workers. Yet for many black and rural Americans living under conditions of racism, poverty, and social isolation, success is difficult to achieve. The competition that results often leads to a deep distrust of others and may pit even close friends and family members against one another on occasion. In a case of magical illness, the most likely attacker is a neighbor, friend, or even a relative with whom the victim is having problems. The most common reasons for magical attacks are arguments within love triangles; family disputes over issues such as child custody, inheritance rights, or living arrangements; and struggles over employment opportunities and finances. Magical attacks in these situations are interpreted as attempts to gain control or advantage over the victim. It is interesting that part of the root doctor's treatment is often some form of family counseling aimed at identifying and solving the social problems that precipitated the magical attack.

In Veronica's case, for example, the root doctor she visited first asked her to tell him about her problems. This somewhat vague and open-ended question did not ask her about illness per se, but rather allowed her to define the parameters of the situation. Veronica did talk about her physical symptoms but she also talked for about thirty minutes about the stresses in her daily life. She told the root doctor, an elderly man who was a lifetime resident of her community, all about her problems finding employment and meeting her family's financial needs. She told him the history of her relationship with Jim and about her efforts to remain on good terms with Jim's family. At the end of her long recitation, the root doctor asked Veronica to tell him what she thought had caused her illness. At that point Veronica described how she began by assuming it was a natural problem. She told him about the different remedies she had tried without success and finally presented to him the evidence that led her to conclude she had been hexed by Jim's girlfriend.

The root doctor then asked Veronica's mother and neighbor, who had accompanied her on the visit, if they agreed. Each one spoke about the situation and why they thought the girlfriend was responsible. At the end of an hour, the root doctor made his diagnosis. He told Veronica she had been hexed by the girlfriend who was jealous of her and her relationship to Jim. He suggested that Veronica was afraid that Jim would forget her and quit supporting the child. Veronica nodded her head in agreement. The root doctor then told her that what she needed to do was take precautions against the evil thoughts of the girlfriend. He recommended that Veronica first tell Jim's mother about the situation so that she could look out for her son. He then told Veronica she needed to use some charms he would give her to protect herself and her child. Finally, he suggested that Veronica quit worrying about Jim because the more she worried, the more she suffered. He concluded by suggesting that maybe it was time Veronica herself began to go out with men again. He said then her mind wouldn't be so focused on Jim and in the meantime she might meet a nice man who could help her out. Veronica's mother agreed with the root doctor and, encouraged, thanked him for pointing this out to Veronica. He then ended the session by giving Veronica a potion to drink to remove the hex. He also suggested that she come back again to purchase from him some lucky charms to ward off evil.

Clearly, in this case, the root doctor provided a forum in which Veronica and her family could talk about their interpersonal stresses and problems. Veronica could voice her fears about losing her child's father to another woman and also express some ambivalence and even guilt over these feelings. Veronica's mother could indicate that she thought Veronica was too obsessed with Jim and needed to get on with life. And, finally, when the root doctor repeated back this notion as advice, Veronica herself was able to accept it.

In many cases I observed, the root doctor elicited family discussion on interpersonal problems. The diagnosis of illness from symptoms was not a significant part of such encounters. Rather, the root doctors allowed the patients themselves to define their problems and even suggest solutions. Frequently, the healer's role appeared to be one of providing validation and authority for the actions suggested initially by the patients themselves. In these instances the actual practice of magical rituals was not emphasized. For the most part, it was the older root doctors who were established residents of local communities and who knew most of the local inhabitants that performed this type of counseling. I also interviewed a few "new" root doctors who were generally younger men who had recently come into a community after living outside the region. These younger root doctors focused more exclusively on magic and employed a variety of showy tricks and spells to dazzle clients who usually requested their help in securing financial gain, bewitching errant lovers, or obtaining revenge on enemies. All of the root doctors I interviewed charged for their services, but the charges varied. Many of the older, resident practitioners charged modest fees for consultation ($5–10) and additional small amounts for medicines and charms. They sometimes even consulted for free if a person could not pay. On the other hand, some of the younger, more magically oriented ones reportedly charged as much as $1,500 for a spell.

Conflicting Expectations and Miscommunication in the Clinical Encounter

The adherents of the rootwork system tend to self-diagnose the nature of illness when it first occurs. This judgment about the nature and severity of the condition suffered leads to treatment choices. In the rootwork system, however, diagnostic decisions are not made solely upon an evaluation of symptoms or signs. Rather the signs of illness are used by people to arrive at a determination of causal etiology. Once cause at the ultimate level (that is, the determination of natural versus unnatural and mind versus body condition) is made, then an appropriate treatment alternative is selected. Thus, when these individuals elect to see physicians, they do so for specific reasons—either because they are suffering from particularly serious or acute natural body problems or because their illnesses have failed to respond to other types of treatment—and consequently they enter the medical encounter with specific expectations. The potential for misunderstandings between these patients and health care providers are multiple.

For example, physicians routinely ask patients in initial medical interviews to report on what is wrong in terms of symptoms. Individuals who accept the principles of the rootwork system, however, often answer the question of what is wrong by naming a particular folk illness category without mentioning specific symptoms. Thus, when the physician attempts to elicit further information on the nature, intensity, and location of the major symptom and other associated ones, the patients perceive the questions to be irrelevant and frequently answer by giving information designed to justify to the physician the reasons why they know themselves to be suffering from a particular folk complaint. To the physician, of course, this information is virtually useless in making a physical diagnosis. Hence both parties frequently become frustrated and the interaction between them may be terminated quickly.

The following example from a clinic encounter in a hospital in the piedmont region of North Carolina illustrates this problem. In this case, a forty-five-year-old black woman had come to the emergency room for treatment, and after an initial interview, had been referred to the internal medicine clinic. The initial interview in this clinic went as follows:

> Physician: What seems to be the trouble, Mrs. Evans?
>
> Patient: Well, Doctor, I've been feelin' poorly with the low blood these days.
>
> Physician: Well, what exactly seems to be the problem?
>
> Patient: Well, Doctor, you see since I lost so much blood five years ago when I lost the baby, I never been the same. It's jus' times like these when things are gettin' next to me that it brings on the spells and my blood gets lower.
>
> Physician: How do you feel? Do you have any pain, does anything hurt?
>
> Patient: Well, you know, not really. But it's jus' the old low blood acting up. I been feelin' kind of logey.

The physician proceeds trying to elicit a chief complaint, and the patient's daughter, who has been sitting in on the interview, tells him that her mother's blood is low. In his frustration with such a vague report, the physician ends up listing "patient feels tired" as the chief complaint and sends the woman off for a series of blood tests. The woman is reluctant to let the nurse take her blood as the following conversation reveals:

Daughter: What are you goin' to do there? What's that needle for?

Nurse: We are just going to take a little blood sample to run some tests and see if your mother's blood is anemic.

Patient: I don't want you takin' no blood.

Nurse: Don't worry, it won't hurt. I'll put on this tube around your arm after I take your pressure. Then it won't hurt. It will just take a second.

Patient: No, you don't need my blood. I done told the doctor that I've been feelin' logey. Why can't he jus' give me something for the low blood so we can go on home?

Nurse: Well, he needs to find out if there is anything wrong with your blood first. It could be you are just a little tired.

Daughter: My mother is just having a bout of low blood. She gets that way every now and then. She don't need a test to tell her that. What do you do with that blood anyway?

Nurse: We examine it to see if there are any problems.

Daughter: But then what do you do with it?

Nurse: What do you mean?

Daughter: Where does it go? Do you keep it for experiments?

Nurse: (Laughing) Oh no, we throw it out. We don't do experiments on people's blood without their permission.

Patient: But if you throw it out, anyone could get a hold of it.

Daughter: Yeah, how do you get rid of it? Do you leave it in the garbage for anyone to get?

Nurse: No, we put it all together and a special company picks it up every afternoon to dispose of it.

Patient: But then it is around all day just sitting back there. Anyone could get it.

At this point, the nurse was summoned to take a phone call for the attending physician. The daughter turned to her mother and suggested that they leave. She said, "Let's get out of here. They aren't goin' to give you what you need. And I don't like this idea of them takin' your blood. Let's go and we'll just see how you're feelin' in a few days. Maybe we can get Dr. Jenkins (a retired family physician in their community) to take a look at you. We'll jus' tell him 'bout the run around we got here." At that point they left, telling the nurse who had returned that they couldn't stay that day because their ride was leaving. After their departure, the nurse commented on how unreliable "those people" (that is, lower-class, black patients) were.

A review of the encounter, however, illustrates several points at which clashing expectations led to miscommunication between the parties involved. Initially, the physician attempted to elicit from the patient a chief complaint in the form of symptomatic information. But then he was presented, instead, with information about a specific folk disorder—that of "low blood." The nature of the response, however, is not readily apparent to people unfamiliar with the ethnomedical system under consideration because the term itself, low blood, appears to describe a symptomatic condition—that is, that of having low blood as in low blood pressure. A common practice in the ethnomedical system, however, involves the use of key symptoms of folk illnesses in the labeling of the category. Thus "low blood" refers not only to the character of the blood as low or bitter, but also stands for a whole host of additional symptoms that comprise the folk disease of low blood. These include lassitude (feeling logey), constipation, weakness, fainting spells, loss of appetite, and general disinterest in one's surroundings. Some or all of these symptoms may be present in a person suffering from low blood. The patient in this encounter, however, does not report on the symptoms initially and eventually does so only reluctantly. Her main concern, having presented her self-diagnosis, is to justify to the physician how she knows it to be so—that is, due to a loss of blood suffered during a miscarriage five years previously. This seemingly irrelevant statement takes on meaning only when one knows the theory operating behind the folk belief, namely that an imbalance in the blood (caused in this case by blood loss) can make the blood either too high and sweet or too low and bitter, thereby resulting in illness.

Physicians often logically assume that patients stating the labels for folk illnesses are in fact reporting symptoms, because folk illness categories in the rootwork system usually are labeled with the name of a specific symptom. The process of labeling the whole with the name of one of its parts is known in linguistics as metonomy. Metonymic labeling is based on a contextual association between two elements. Thus cold, for example, refers in a literal sense to a physical state of lacking heat. When we say that someone has "caught cold," however, we are emphasizing the fact that the physical state of "cold" may either cause, or be associated with, certain respiratory complaints which, as illness entities, we often label and call "colds." In the metonymic labeling process, therefore, the particular parts we use to stand for and label the category are usually those with some special significance for us.

The process of labeling a disease category with the term for a key symptom is common across all cultures. The particular symptoms chosen to name illnesses, however, are usually significant in one of three ways. Some symptoms are used to label illness categories because the presence of the symptom marks the onset of the illness. The presence of measles or of pox, for instance, marks the onset of the diseases known by those names. Other symptoms may be chosen as labels for illness because they are believed to be instrumental in causing the illness condition. Low blood or a lack of blood, for example, is believed to cause the group of symptoms associated with disease labeled, "low blood." Finally, certain symptoms may be used to name an illness category because they are especially salient or because they are thought to be especially characteristic of a particular illness. This latter process occurs frequently in the labeling of magical, rootwork conditions. "Paralysis or fading," for example, is a category of magical illness that includes the symptoms of numbness in the feet, legs, hands, and arms; a lack of interest in daily life; loss of appetite; dysphasia; loss of memory; and/or impotence in males. If the condition worsens, afflicted individuals believe they will eventually become paralyzed and hence be unable to walk and function in daily life. Thus "paralysis" is an especially salient or focal symptom for the illness and is used to label it, but the symptom itself may not be present at the onset of the illness. So when a patient tells a physician, "I'm paralyzed," he is not necessarily saying that he cannot walk in a literal sense. Rather, by saying "I'm paralyzed," or "I'm fading," the individual is signaling the presence of a particular ethnomedical complaint.

Metonymic labeling occurs frequently in Western medicine as well, but physicians are not confused by it because they are familiar with the disease categories and associated symptoms. The confusion emerges when patient terms label ethnomedical categories that are not generally known to health care providers.

A second source of difficulty in the clinic encounter recounted above emerges from the differential expectations of the participants. The patient has decided in advance that she is suffering from a natural, body problem labeled low blood. She tells this to the physician and expects that he will act on the information to prescribe immediately the appropriate medicine to correct the condition, a medicine that will "sweeten" or "build up" the blood. When he calls, instead, for blood tests to determine the nature of the problem, the patient feels resentful because her self-diagnosis has been questioned and her justifying information rejected. I interviewed this patient after the reported encounter and she said that she felt the doctor was "jus' a young one who didn't really know nothin' 'bout sickness. 'Cause if he did, he would've given me my medicines then and there without all that foolishness." The resident, however, had a different impression of the encounter. He told it this way: "I just don't understand some of the people we get in here. They can't tell you what's wrong with them, and they don't want to hear what you have to say. I think most of it is in their minds anyway. Why do you think they left like that? They just wanted to talk, but when it came time for the needle, they had had enough. The problem is that we waste a lot of time and money on people like that who don't really want or need help." The nurse did not come to the same conclusion about the patients as the resident did. She thought, instead, that the patient and her daughter were just "poor, country folks" who didn't understand how medicine worked. She thought they were frightened about giving blood and left before they could be convinced of the need to take the test. But then, giving voice to her own stereotypes, the nurse added, "What difference does it make anyway. When you try to help these people, they don't follow through. You give them medicine and they don't take it right, or they don't take it at all. They never come back for follow-up appointments, and you won't see them again until they get very sick."

So why did the two women leave before completing the blood tests? Their version of the situation was quite different, as the daughter explained:

> I don't like the idea of my Mother giving her blood to them. You heard the nurse. She don't know what's gonna happen to that blood. They take it and look at it. Then they'll jus' tell you that you ain't got nothin'. But while you're there foolin' around, where does your blood go? Anybody could get a hold of it. And then where would you be? A body's got to be careful. We knows some of the people that work in that place, and what if one of them was to see us there. No tellin' what could happen to that blood. You gots to be careful.

In other words, blood is a powerful life substance that could be used in magical spells to harm a person. Letting someone take your blood is an act of trust, and obviously these two patients did not trust the medical staff to safeguard the blood, especially when they were not convinced that the test was necessary in the first place.

The Influence of Traditional Beliefs on Patterns of Illness Decisionmaking

A key feature of most ethnomedical systems is the pluralistic nature of treatment choice. Adherents of the rootwork system, for example, often seek mainstream medical care for natural body problems and may also end up in clinics and hospitals seeking treatment for magical illnesses. The implications of pluralistic use patterns for patient compliance with mainstream care are illustrated in two case studies from eastern North Carolina.

Henry Wilson, a thirty-six-year-old black male, first reported to a local hospital emergency room for treatment for injuries that occurred when he was struck by a car. His chief complaint was of lower back pain and scrapes. He was hospitalized overnight for observation and released the next day with a prescription for pain pills. Upon his return home, his condition failed to improve, and he sought the advice of his mother. She began treating him at home with back rubs of hot oil and the application of poultices containing herbs, mustard, and Vicks vapor rub. Henry began to feel some relief and returned to his carpentry job. Two weeks later he was seen again in the emergency room for a work-related injury to his hand. A doctor stitched his hand, prescribed an antibiotic, and sent him home. He began to recover, but within two weeks had begun to experience back pain again. Henry became increasingly worried because he had a numb feeling in his right leg—"as if it was going to sleep." He found no relief with his medicines or mother's home remedies, and at her suggestion went to see a local herbalist.

The feeling failed to go away, and Henry's mother suggested he go back to the hospital. He refused and returned to work instead. About a month later, the numb sensation became more pronounced and spread to both legs. Henry spoke to a friend about it who suggested that maybe the illness was unrelated to his other problems and was instead the result of a hex cast by an ex-girlfriend. The friend reminded Henry that his ex-girlfriend had been very angry over their breakup and had threatened him that he would be sorry about it one day. Henry scoffed at the idea of a hex but by the next morning he could not walk. His mother called an ambulance and took him to the emergency room. This time he was referred to Neurology and given a complete workup. The physicians could find no physical cause for his paralysis. In the meantime, Henry's mother made inquiries about the ex-girlfriend and determined that she had probably put a hex on her son. She convinced Henry to leave the hospital and see a root doctor. The root doctor confirmed the hex and gave Henry a potion to remove it. Henry reported a complete recovery after the visit and resolved to be more careful, "about who I take up with" in the future.

The case of Inez Perry, a twenty-six-year-old black woman, illustrates a different pattern of pluralistic use. Inez suffered a miscarriage in the fourth month of her pregnancy. She went to the emergency room of the local hospital where she was attended and released with a follow-up appointment in the OB-GYN outpatient clinic the next day. Inez did not show up for her appointment, and the medical personnel lost track of her case. When questioned about why she missed her appointment, Inez reported dissatisfaction with the hospital personnel who, she said, never told her what was going on. She returned home from that visit and continued for two weeks to suffer intermittent bleeding, cramps, and a feeling of listlessness and depression. Her aunt made her herbal teas and recruited a neighbor woman to give her massages. Although Inez reported some relief, she continued to feel listless and depressed.

At this point, her aunt decided that she was suffering emotionally from her sins. Her aunt told how Inez had been seeing a married man and had conceived the child. Because the man refused to leave his wife, the aunt concluded that her niece had subconsciously wished to abort the child—a sin in God's eyes. She told Inez that the miscarriage was a punishment sent by God and convinced her to see the minister at the Holiness Church for help. Inez went with her aunt to talk with the minister. She reported that the minister persuaded her to confess in an emotional scene in which she cried, convulsed, and was "touched by the hand of God." At that point, Inez says she felt the misery and pain leave her body and felt herself made whole again. Accepted into the church the next week, Inez began to become active in the religion and severed her relationship with the married man. She vowed that in the future she would take all of her problems to the Lord first because, "He is all-powerful; His medicine is the only medicine I need."

In each of these cases, the patients are using a number of very different treatment alternatives, often simultaneously. The ways that they conceptualize illness and the therapies they embrace have consequences for their adherence to mainstream practices. In the first case study one man has, over the course of six weeks, seen a physician three times, used a variety of home and over-the-counter remedies, consulted with a herbalist, and seen a root doctor for what he sees to be a related sequence of events. This bewildering variety of choices reflects a seemingly random pattern of behavior that may prove incomprehensible to mainstream practitioners who have no understanding of the attributions of disease causation and assessments of treatment efficacy in the ethnomedical system. A problem originally classified as natural became reclassified over time and connected to other, seemingly accidental events, as part of an unnatural disorder caused by a spell. The magical attribution provides meaning to the misfortunes suffered by the man and gives him an avenue to put an end to his misfortunes. Once he does so, the physical symptoms of paralysis disappear.

In the second case, a woman enters the medical system for an emergency miscarriage. The physician handles her physical discomfort but does not attempt to "tell her what is going on" by discussing the loss itself. Thus, she is left with the emotional pain and guilt to resolve. This takes place in the religious sphere where personal counseling and forgiveness allow her to put an end to a difficult time in her life and move forward free of physical and emotional symptoms.

In large part the effectiveness and persistence of ethnomedical beliefs and practices stem from their ability to provide answers that people need to the larger questions raised by illness. When a patient wants to know why me, what caused my illness, why is it happening now, and how can I cure it, scientific explanations may not be enough. All people want comfort, answers to unanswerable questions, and some assurance that illness can be treated effectively. For many of the South's rural poor, illness also signals a cry for social and emotional support by those who can no longer cope with the burdens of a difficult life under conditions of uncertainty. Such support is not usually provided by the mainstream medical system. So while patients may turn to physicians for physical relief, they are more likely to look to ministers, neighbors, friends, and rootworkers to provide social healing and a sense of mastery and control over life.

Conclusion

Health professionals working in the rural South will probably encounter patients in the mainstream system who simultaneously hold traditional ethnomedical beliefs. These beliefs are likely to shape the patient's pattern of illness decisionmaking and treatment choice, expectations of the clinical encounter, and presentation of symptoms. An awareness of and respect for these traditional beliefs will facilitate the mainstream provider's ability to work with such patients effectively. A realization, for example, that patients may use multiple providers simultaneously means that compliance with mainstream treatment regimes cannot be taken for granted. The concerned practitioner can, as Peter Lichstein demonstrates in chapter six, elicit such information from the patient and use it in negotiating a joint therapeutic plan.

Similarly, an awareness of the structure of ethnomedical beliefs can enable practitioners to predict and prepare for the possibility of conflicting expectations in the clinical encounter. Adherents of rootwork possess a set of ethnomedical illness categories that are labeled and defined differently from those of mainstream medicine. The practitioner who realizes this can avoid the confusion that results when such illness labels are mistaken for symptom reports.

Finally, the practitioner can use ethnomedical information to aid in delineating the goals of the patient in the medical encounter. The rootwork adherent enters the mainstream system with well-defined notions about the type of illness suffered and the treatment desired. The health practitioner needs to begin the patient session by eliciting such information in order to establish a basis from which to work with the patient in negotiating shared treatment goals.

Success in resolving cultural differences is ultimately dependent on sensitivity to, and respect for, alternative systems of belief about health and disease. Respect, however, does not necessarily mean approval. Physicians need to know what their patients believe about illness in order to work with them more effectively. But, as Peter Lichstein points out in chapter six, physicians do not necessarily need to adopt ethnomedical labels or attempt to emulate ethnomedical practices to be successful in treating illnesses in traditional populations. Ultimately, each case is unique, and the plans developed by clinicians to deal with such cases will be too. The success achieved, however, will always be a measure of the rapport established between the people involved. An awareness and understanding of different cultural traditions is an important first step in the development of such rapport.

Notes

1. This essay draws on fieldwork conducted in piedmont and coastal communities of North Carolina. Interviews with the rural elderly on alternative health care use in ten counties in

eastern North Carolina were funded by a grant from the Agency for Health Care Policy and Research carried out jointly with Jim Mitchell of the East Carolina University Center on Aging. The tables included in this article are reprinted with permission from a 1987 article in the *Southern Medical Journal.* Informants' names, with the exception Mrs. Emma Dupree, have been changed in the text to protect their confidentiality. Titles are used with names when informants specifically preferred to be addressed and referred to in that manner. I thank Ronald Hoag and two anonymous reviewers for comments on an earlier version of this paper and Virginia Nichols for suggesting the title.

2. I am indebted to a reviewer of this manuscript who pointed out that the word "hex" comes from a German root word introduced into the U.S. vocabulary around 1930 through a hex murder in York County, Pennsylvania. This would suggest that the term is a late loan in the North Carolina vocabulary and although it is widely used by my informants, there is no documented evidence of the use of this term before the twentieth century.

References

Baldwin, Karen. "Mrs. Emma Dupree: 'That Little Medicine Thing'." *North Carolina Folklore Journal* 32.2 (1984): 50–53.

Campinha-Bacote, Josepha. "Culturological Assessment: An Important Factor in Psychiatric Consultation-Liaison Nursing." *Archives of Psychiatric Nursing* 2.4 (1988): 244–50.

Cappannari, Stephen C., Bruce Rau, Harry S. Abram, and Denton C. Buchanan. "Voodoo in the General Hospital—A Case of Hexing and Regional Enteritis." *Journal of the American Medical Association* 232.9 (1975): 938–40.

Dupree, Emma Mrs., personal interview, July 7, 1990.

Foster, George M., and Barbara G. Anderson. *Medical Anthropology.* New York: John Wiley and Sons, 1978.

Freemon, Frank R., M.D., and Frank T. Drake, M.D. "Abnormal Emotional Reactions to Hospitalization Jeopardizing Medical Treatment." *Psychosomatics* 8 (1967): 150–55.

Golden, Kenneth M. "Voodoo in Africa and the United States." *American Journal of Psychiatry* 134.12 (1977): 1,425–27.

Gums, John G., and Deborah Stier Carson. "Influence of Folk Medicine on the Family Practitioner." *Southern Medical Journal* 80.2 (1987): 209–12.

Hall, Arthur L., and Peter G. Bourne. "Indigenous Therapists in a Southern Black Community." *Archives of General Psychiatry* 28 (1973): 137–42.

Hill, Carole E. "A Folk Medical System in the American South: Some Practical Considerations." *Southern Medical Journal* 64 (1977): 11–17.

Hill, Carole E., and Holly F. Mathews. "Traditional Health Beliefs and Practices among Southern Rural Blacks: A Complement to Biomedicine." *Perspectives on the American South.* Ed. Merle Black and John S. Reed. New York: Gordon and Breach, 1981. 307–22.

Hillard, James R., and Kenneth Rockwell. "Dysesthesia, Witchcraft and Conversion Reactions: A Case Successfully Treated with Psychotherapy." *Journal of the American Medical Association* 240.16 (1978): 1,742–44.

Jackson, Bruce E. "The Other Kind of Doctor: Conjure and Magic in Black American Folk Medicine." *American Folk Medicine: A Symposium.* Ed. Wayland D. Hand. Berkeley: University of California Press, 1976. 259–72.

Jaeckle, Kurt A., M.D., and Frank R. Freemon, M.D. "Pokeweed Poisoning." *Southern Medical Journal* 74.5 (1981): 639–40.

Jordan, W. C. "Voodoo Medicine." *Textbook of Black-Related Diseases.* Ed. Richard Allen Williams. New York: McGraw-Hill, 1975. 716–38.

Kimball, Chase Patterson. "A Case of Pseudocyesis Caused by 'Roots'." *American Journal of Obstetrical Gynecology* 107 (1976): 801–3.

Levine, Lawrence W. *Black Culture and Black Consciousness.* New York: Oxford University Press, 1977.

McCall, G. J. "Symbiosis: The Case of Hoodoo and the Numbers Racket." *Social Forces* 10 (1963): 361–71.

Maduro, J. R. J. "Hoodoo Possession in San Francisco: Notes on the Therapeutic Aspects of Regression." *Ethos* 3 (1975): 425–27.

Malinowski, Bronislaw. *Magic, Science and Religion, and Other Essays.* Boston: Beacon, 1948.

Mathews, Holly F. "Rootwork: Description of an Ethnomedical System in the American South." *Southern Medical Journal* 80.7 (1987): 885–91.

Moerman, Daniel E. "High-low, Bitter-sweet: An American Folk Medical System." *Proceedings of the Central States Anthropological Society* 1 (1975): 47–50.

Pockrein, G. A. "Humoralism and Social Development in Colonial America." *Journal of the American Medical Association* 245.17 (1981): 1,755–57.

Saphir, J. Robin, Arnold Gold, James Giambrone, and James F. Holland. "Voodoo Poisoning in Buffalo, New York." *Journal of the American Medical Association* 202 (1967): 437–38.

Savitt, Todd L. *Medicine and Slavery.* Urbana: University of Illinois Press, 1978.

Little Medicine Thing: Mrs. Emma Dupree, dir. Walter Shepherd and James Young, Office of Health Services Research and Development, East Carolina University School of Medicine, 1980.

Snow, Loudell F. "Folk Beliefs and Their Implications for Care of Patients—A Review Based on Studies among Black Americans." *Annals of Internal Medicine* 81 (1974): 82–96.

———. "Popular Medicine in a Black Neighborhood." *Ethnic Medicine in the Southwest.* Ed. E. H. Spicer. Tucson: University of Arizona Press, 1977. 19–95.

———. "Sorcerers, Saints and Charlatans: Black Folk Healers in Urban America." *Culture, Medicine and Psychiatry* 2 (1978): 69–106.

———. "Traditional Health Beliefs and Practices among Lower Class Black Americans." *Western Journal of Medicine* 139 (1983): 820–28.

Tallant, R. *Voodoo in New Orleans.* New York: Macmillan, 1946.

Tinling, David C. "Voodoo, Root Work, and Medicine." *Psychosomatic Medicine* 29.5 (1967): 483–90.

Wallis, R., and Peter Morley. "Introduction." *Marginal Medicine.* Ed. R. Wallis and Peter Morley. New York: Free, 1976. 9–19.

Whitten, Norman E. "Contemporary Patterns of Malign Occultism among Negros in North Carolina." *Journal of American Folklore* 75.298 (1962): 311–25.

Wintrob, Ronald M. "The Influence of Others: Witchcraft and Rootwork and Explanations of Behavior Differences." *Journal of Nervous and Mental Disease* 156.5 (1973): 318–26.

6. Rootwork from the Clinician's Perspective

Peter R. Lichstein

Physicians who treat patients from diverse cultural backgrounds face challenges rarely discussed in medical education. This essay will address some of the questions raised when a patient who believes he or she has been hexed or made ill by rootwork goes to the physician's office or the hospital. In these settings, cases of hexing invariably provoke feelings of fascination, anxiety, and uncertainty in the medical staff. They provide ample evidence that our patients' beliefs about illness and medical care frequently differ from the biotechnical explanations of modern medical practice.

Cases of hexing are instructive for the light they shed on the ways in which patients experience and interpret symptoms, as well as how and from whom they seek medical care. Epidemiologic studies have documented that between 75 and 90 percent of illness episodes are treated outside the established medical care system (Eisenberg 1980, 279). Most illnesses are self-treated at home. Some patients seek care from nonphysician alternatives such as a chiropractor, a pharmacist, or a folk health practitioner. The patient's beliefs influence decisions about how serious a symptom is and whether or not it represents a threat to the individual's current and future well-being and are critical determinants of illness behavior (Zola 218).

The patient's beliefs about illness often lack formal organization or consistency; they may be fluid, changing with time and circumstance. One patient may subscribe to a variety of beliefs, some medical, others from folk or personal systems, and may shift from one belief to another without experiencing cognitive dissonance or feeling troubled by the apparent contradictions. Health care may be sought from a variety of practitioners, each treating the patient from a unique perspective. Therefore, it cannot be assumed that patients with folk medical beliefs seek care only from folk medical practitioners. These patients come to physicians with surprising frequency, although they rarely talk about or share their beliefs.

Frequently the beliefs of an individual patient do not conform with the anthropologist's description of generally held beliefs in the community. Overreliance on stereotypical descriptions may lead to prejudice and inaccurate assumptions about what a patient thinks and how he or she will behave. Each patient's response to illness reflects a unique blend of cultural, familial, and personal influences and experiences. It is the clinician's task to approach each new patient with an open mind, seeking to understand the various explanatory models by which the patient lives, experiences, and acts. By failing to do so, a decisive element in the patient's care may be overlooked. For example, the doctor may try to treat symptoms with medications which, because of his or her beliefs, the patient never takes.

Illness provokes a variety of cognitive and emotional reactions, some adaptive and some not. Patients often feel helpless and confused and cut off from their communities and families. Although the practice of rootwork, described by Holly Mathews in chapter five, may seem bizarre, it can be viewed as an explanatory model that helps individuals and communities cope with the anxieties and uncertainties of sickness. At times of illness, patients try to find answers to questions such as, "Why me?" "Why now?" "What have I done to deserve this?" "What should I do?" and "What will become of me?" Illness beliefs provide a structure for answering these and other questions. They help the patient find meaning in sickness. In fact, most visits to physicians, excluding those for major trauma or critical illness, are motivated in part by requests for interpretation of symptoms (Eisenberg 1981, 245). The doctor's task is to help bring order to the chaos of illness.

The comfort provided by a cognitive model is, in large part, independent of its scientific validity. The model must make sense to the patient, provide a course of action with merits that the patient can understand, and help the patient establish healing relationships with others. Although the biotechnical approach of modern medicine may be scientifically valid, its perspective is often narrowly focused on the control of disease through technical means. All symptoms are viewed as the manifestation of disease processes that alter the structure or function of bodily tissues and organs. The biotechnical model does not value an understanding of the patient's lived world. It fails to address the patient's need for meaning and restored relationships and employs a language system that may mystify rather than inform. Like all belief systems, the biotechnical approach is value laden and culturally determined (Engel 130).

Bridging the cultural gap that separates and frequently alienates doctor and patient requires a blend of intellectual flexibility and nonjudgmental openness. The doctor's vision must expand beyond the medicocentric to creatively weave the patient's explanatory model into the fabric of care. At the technologic-folk interface the physician must actively inquire about the patient's beliefs and negotiate a shared approach to diagnosis and therapy (Weimer and Mintz 359). In return for these efforts, the physician learns how the patient's beliefs modify his or her interpretation of symptoms, guide decisions that determine when and from whom care is sought, and shape the patient's response to suffering and disability. With this knowledge, a therapeutic plan that helps the patient find meaning and restored relationships, in addition to the benefits of biotechnical care, becomes a realistic goal. Although this chapter deals specifically with the folk practice of rootwork, similar principles may be applied to all patients. Even the most sophisticated patient, when under stress and threatened by sickness or disability, may turn in the quest for meaning to magical or primitive ideas acquired from family and community. Finding a common language is a central task for many clinical encounters.

The following case examples illustrate problems that arise when the cultural framework of the physician and patient differs; when they are geographically close, yet culturally distant. In these cases, the physician's role as interpreter is complex and challenging.[1]

Case One

B.L., a fifty-five-year-old married black woman, was brought to the hospital with intermittent fever, weight loss, fatigue, and pain in her joints. Her primary care physicians were puzzled by her complex symptoms and described her as a "strange lady." She spent most of the day lying in bed, her back turned to her doctors, and she answered questions in monosyllables. No one had been able to establish rapport with her, and no one had elicited a detailed history.

The author was asked to help with the evaluation of her anemia. He had recently read David C. Tinling's review of seven cases of hexing in a northern city. Tinling alerts physicians that a belief in rootwork is not uncommon and that although most patients want to talk about being hexed, they are frequently reluctant to do so for fear of being ridiculed or misunderstood (489). The author wondered if this woman's withdrawal might stem from her beliefs about illness. Cultural barriers might cause her fear and uncertainty in the modern hospital. In this setting Tinling encourages physicians to be active during the interview, asking questions and using the patient's own language as much as possible. When this patient was asked if she thought "roots" might be involved in her case, there was an abrupt change in her behavior. She turned toward her physicians and asked how medical doctors knew about roots. She wondered if medical doctors could remove the hex but remained suspicious that they would be powerless or perhaps do her harm if they tried.

Once the barriers to communication were breached, she became a willing historian and far more involved in her medical workup. Her experiences with rootwork dated from her childhood in the Piedmont of North Carolina. She remembered hearing about "snakes coming out of peoples' arms" and people made sick or well by magic. Her current illness began two months earlier when she felt "run down" and "aching all over." Her family physician diagnosed her condition as a bad cold and prescribed an antibiotic. He reassured her that her laboratory tests were normal. Continuing to feel poorly despite the medication, she consulted a neighbor who "knew a lot about hexes." From the neighbor she learned that several women in the community were jealous of her good-looking and fully employed husband. The neighbor reported that a "hoodoo man" had been employed to put a "root" on her and that any medicine prescribed by a medical doctor would only make things worse. As in many cases of hexing, jealousy was the motive and the hex was actually placed by a specially hired individual, the root doctor (Snow 86). This patient shared the common belief that only another root doctor could remove the hex but she was unable, or perhaps unwilling, to locate one. She experienced a period of profound helplessness as her symptoms increased. She didn't know where or to whom she could turn. Initially, she refused to go to the hospital for her complaints, fearing that the hex would intensify. Only at her husband's insistence did she reluctantly seek further medical care.

After admission to the hospital she felt isolated and fearful. She doubted the medical staff would understand or accept her belief in hexes, and an atmosphere of confrontation dominated the first hospital days. Feeling uneasy about the care of this difficult patient, her primary care physicians requested multiple consultations from medical specialists. However, when she discovered that physicians were interested in her beliefs and willing to listen to her concerns, she felt more confident in their abilities and became a more cooperative patient.

Subsequent tests revealed that she suffered from systemic lupus erythematosus (SLE), a multisystem inflammatory disease of unknown cause. She was started on prednisone, a medication which lessens the inflammatory process, with gradual improvement in her symptoms. As her faith in the doctors increased and her symptoms decreased, she talked less about hexes, but remained concerned that the medication might work against her as her neighbor predicted. Her doctors explained that the medication would help build her strength so that she could cope with the jealousy of her difficult neighbors. They assured her of their commitment to her care and willingness to discuss her home problems as well as her disease. They carefully avoided denegrating her belief in hexes. Rather, they emphasized that any person who was feeling sick would look for an explanation that made sense to them. They attempted to educate her about the treatment of SLE and how this illness could explain her various symptoms.

Discharged on a maintenance dose of prednisone, she returned to her home, only to experience an abrupt increase in symptoms. Fearing that the hex was causing her decline and remembering what her neighbor had said about the paradoxical effect of medications, she stopped taking the prednisone. Several weeks later she arrived at the hospital by ambulance. Her disease had progressed to a fulminate stage, and she required support in the critical care unit.

This case demonstrates the communication problems that frequently occur when a patient feels isolated by cultural barriers. Like most patients who believe in hexes, she seemed relieved when directly asked about the possibility that "roots" might be causing her symptoms. She responded positively to a nonjudgmental interview style and became a willing historian. Once her beliefs were understood, an approach to her treatment was negotiated. She became an ally in the therapeutic process without loss of personal integrity. Her doctors were able to shift away from a medicocentric point of reference.

Unfortunately, the patient returned to an unchanged community environment and lost contact with her physicians. The psychosocial factors that had initially caused her to delay seeking care were operative once again. She felt that her bodily symptoms were an indicator of interpersonal discord rather than disease. In retrospect, education about the likelihood of a relapse and what to do if it occurred may not have been adequate. Finally, her disease process may have produced emotional problems that increased the patient's vulnerability to beliefs such as rootwork (Kirkpatrick 1,937).

Case Two

Tragic consequences may result if health care beliefs run contrary to the realities of disease and negotiation fails to bridge the cultural gap.

A sixteen-year-old black girl with SLE was diagnosed as suffering from severe inflammation of the heart, lungs, and kidneys. She relied on her parents to bring her to the clinic and frequently missed her appointments. A belief in rootwork dominated the family's approach to this and other illnesses. As a result, their utilization of medical doctors and prescribed medications was episodic and erratic. The patient's condition worsened, and the dose of her medication was increased. However, her doctors feared she was not taking (or being given) her pills. Repeated meetings with the parents left her doctors feeling frustrated. A social worker was sent to investigate the home and assess the safety of the environment. Despite these efforts, the family continued to believe that with time the hex would lift and that medication was really not needed. Her doctors encouraged the family to bring her to the hospital if her condition continued to deteriorate. Despite signs of progressive failure, her parents' belief that only magic would help persisted. They consulted a rootworker in their community, but refused to tell the medical doctors what had been prescribed. Several months later the patient died at home of apparent respiratory failure at the age of eighteen.

Case Three

D.P., a thirty-nine-year-old black woman, was admitted to the hospital with respiratory failure of undetermined etiology. She had a history of hypertension and valvular heart disease, but these problems did not explain the sudden difficulties with breathing. Soon after being removed from the respirator she demanded a hospital discharge and signed out against medical advice. She was readmitted with a similar episode several weeks later. After careful questioning she admitted believing that she had been hexed. She reported feeling poorly for several weeks and, on the advice of friends, went to a rootworker who "knew my problem without me telling him." He knew she was having "twitching in her stomach" and problems with her estranged husband. She found his ability to diagnose her problems with a single glance most impressive. He gave her perfumed oils to put in her bath for nine consecutive nights and "bark" to chew three times a day for the full nine days. Soon after chewing the bark, which she described as bitter, she developed an irritated throat, fever, drowsiness, slow pulse, and progressive shortness of breath. She reported chewing the bark just prior to both hospital admissions. A sample of the bark was identified as deadly nightshade containing the highly toxic compound solanine (Mack 258).

After the second hospitalization her doctors felt that they had educated her regarding the dangers of the bark and impressed her with the need for strict compliance with a medical regimen. A psychiatric consultant found no evidence of an ongoing psychosis or other significant mental disorder. Within several months, however, she developed increasing shortness of breath due to progression of her heart disease. She was admitted to a community hospital and later transferred to our center. The medical intern assigned to her case was aware of the prior history of rootwork. She attempted to bridge the cultural gap by discussing the patient's beliefs and fears. The patient admitted wondering if another root was being worked, causing the current bout of breathlessness. The intern, wishing to reassure the patient, told her that, "If that's what you believe, you might need to find someone who can take the root off." Interpreting this statement to mean that the doctors "wanted" her to resume her prior folk practices the patient called a friend to bring more of the bark to her hospital room. After chewing it she again suffered an episode of respiratory failure requiring her third ICU stay.

This case raises many issues, including the possibility of criminal activity. This woman nearly died from repeated solanine poisoning. The medical staff found it difficult to understand her recurrent bouts of self-inflicted illness. Her allegiance to the rootworker is, in fact, integral to the magical belief system (Snow 93). She considered his ability to diagnose sickness by looking into the patient's eyes a God-given power that could not be matched by medical doctors who must gain their expertise through study. Whether the rootworker was intentionally trying to poison the patient or simply had an inadequate knowledge of the poisonous properties of plants was never determined. Either way, her case highlights the potential dangers of using herbal remedies. It also reminds us of the importance of the words that doctors use with their patients and the need to make communications as clear as possible. The well-meaning intern was unprepared for the extraordinary impact of her words and the near fatal consequences.

Case Four

Cases of suspected hexing often represent the patient's attempt to explain symptoms that are vague, chronic, or unresponsive to medical treatment. In my experience, this is the most common presentation for rootwork beliefs in clinical practice. A belief in magic, perhaps buried since childhood, is activated by the anxiety and uncertainty of illness. This often happens when the physician has not provided the patient with an acceptable explanation for the illness. In these cases the patient rarely reports clear signs that a root has been placed. Rather, the patient experiences a vague foreboding that a root may have been cast.

A sixty-seven-year-old married black woman came to the psychiatric hospital with symptoms of depression and weight loss. Several days later she told a nurse that she thought her illness was caused by a "jinx." Word quickly spread that the patient had peculiar beliefs. Her doctors wondered how to proceed; how to cure a hex. After further questioning, she reported similar episodes of fatigue and depression in the past. The current episode began with unexplained crying spells three months before her admission. When her family physician reported that all of her laboratory tests were normal, the patient began wondering if her illness might be "unnatural" (caused by a root). She felt that "if the good doctor can't find out what's wrong and can't help me, maybe it's a jinx." Using the folk belief system as a way to make sense of symptoms that her physician had been unable to explain, she began looking for signs of a hex and tried to discover who might have worked it and why. She decided that dust under the furniture had been placed there to make her sick and felt that her seat in church had been "dressed" to do her harm. Losing faith in her family and friends and feeling increasingly vulnerable, she felt that "just about anyone might be hurting me."

After reviewing the clinical literature on rootwork and eliciting a more detailed description of the patient's experiences, the staff decided that her belief in hexing was not in itself a disease; therefore, it did not require cure. It seemed that activation of a latent belief system learned during childhood expressed underlying feelings of helplessness in the face of continuing symptoms that had not been explained or relieved. By exploring her sense of social isolation, sadness, and persecution, the staff directed the patient's attention toward her real-life problems with her husband and their home finances. Her doctors had reassured her that they had encountered and been able to help other patients who felt they had been hexed. She seemed pleased that the doctors would work with, rather than against her beliefs, even though they disclaimed any special or magical powers. In fact, her doctors explicitly stated that they would not be employing magic in her care.

With time, she talked less about hexes and more about troubles at home. To counter her fear that the jinx left her powerless, the resources of the therapeutic hospital community and the patient's personal ability to overcome evil were emphasized. Discussions of practical strategies for coping with problems became the focus of her treatment. Since she remembered that "potions" could help with hexes, she was prescribed a multivitamin elixir to help "build up her strength," in addition to antidepressant medication. She was educated about how an "imbalance" in brain chemistry can lead to depression and that medication can bring the person back into balance. Gradually her mood and social functioning improved, although if questioned directly she retained her belief in hexing. She was discharged with a diagnosis of recurrent major depressive illness.

The medical staff's initial anxiety and uncertainty when faced with a case of hexing is typical of the technologic-folk interface (Lyles and Hillard 663). With this case, the staff was caught off guard and had not as yet formulated a diagnostic or therapeutic plan. Several staff members reported seeing physicians remove hexes by giving medications that induced flushing, vomiting, diarrhea, or a change in urine color, administered with a strong verbal suggestion that "when the medicine works, the hex will be gone." Similar benefits can usually be obtained without purposeful deception. Careful attention to the patient's history, combined with a basic knowledge of cultural beliefs, promoted an empathic doctor-patient relationship and a happy outcome. The treatment honored and protected the integrity of the patient and her physician. It focused on helping the patient return to adaptive responses to life problems rather than discrediting her beliefs and the role they played in her world view.

Case Five

Some patients believe that only a root doctor can remove the hex. It has been suggested that in these cases the medical physicians may refer the patient to a traditional practitioner (Weimer and Mintz 360). This case highlights potential pitfalls of this approach if undertaken without adequate communication between medical and traditional healers.

A twenty-year-old black female college student was hospitalized for increasingly bizarre behavior. Usually a good student, her grades had deteriorated and she was arrested for erratic driving. She believed that her symptoms resulted from a "root" placed by her college roommate. As evidence she described a pair of white shoes, given to her by her mother, that had been stolen and used to work a "spell" on her. She also believed that her roommate had obtained "powders" from a root doctor and that her poisoned food now tasted "funny." The initial differential diagnosis included schizophrenia, manic depressive illness, or a possible drug intoxication. Her medical evaluation was unremarkable and she was given a tentative diagnosis of an acute functional psychosis.

Throughout her brief hospitalization, the patient and her family insisted that her symptoms were caused by a hex and not by mental illness. They believed that only a root doctor could cure her. After her symptoms had improved considerably with antipsychotic medication, the doctors decided to let her leave the hospital to seek consultation with a root doctor known to the family. It was hoped that the family would appreciate this flexibility and respect for traditional beliefs and that a more trusting relationship would eventually develop. A follow-up visit was scheduled for continued treatment.

Soon after discharge, the patient visited a root doctor, who apparently instructed her to discontinue her medications and begin a series of ritual baths, Bible readings, and administration of a nicotine-containing "potion." Within one week she was readmitted to the hospital with increased agitation. Therapeutic efforts during the second hospitalization centered on problems at home and conflicts with her parents. Her symptoms decreased and she was discharged on lithium carbonate for manic depressive illness.

In retrospect, it appeared that the family utilized their belief in rootwork to deny the diagnosis of mental illness. From a cultural perspective, it was more acceptable to label the daughter "hexed" than "crazy" (Snow 86). The medical staff's efforts to support cultural traditions and avoid confrontation had backfired. The root doctor sabotaged their efforts. Collaboration between medical and traditional healers must include shared goals and therapies that are acceptable to both parties. Referral to a root doctor whom the physician does not know is fraught with peril. Successful applications of combined traditional and biotechnical therapies, as reported on American Indian reservations and in Africa, depend on explicitly shared goals between practitioners. Communication with the traditional practitioner is essential.

This case provides several additional perspectives on rootwork. The root had worked through the principles of contagious and sympathetic magic. The patient believed that substances were placed in her food to affect her body (contagious magic) and items of clothing, the white shoes, were used to influence her from afar (sympathetic magic) (Snow 85). She was the object of disapproval in a family that tried to avoid outright contention. It has been proposed that in the appropriate sociocultural context this type of family may single out one member—usually a woman—as vulnerable to a hex (Leininger 77). Furthermore, psychiatric conditions may provide the heightened suggestibility linked to the phenomenon of witchcraft in the Middle Ages, although social factors may be more decisive (Spanos 421). It certainly cannot be assumed that all patients who believe in hexing are mentally ill. Since it is often difficult to determine if bizarre illness beliefs represent shared cultural ideas or personalized delusions caused by a psychiatric disorder, a psychiatric consultant may be helpful in the diagnostic process.

Case Six

Frequently the patient's belief in rootwork is never revealed to the physician. The following case illustrates that a patient can receive intensive medical therapy from physicians who are unaware of what is going on in the patient's mind. They had observed the patient's behavior and knew what he said but not what he thought. It is fascinating and humbling how little we know about some of our patients.

A black male in his mid-sixties was hospitalized for difficulty with swallowing. Carcinoma of the esophagus was diagnosed and he underwent an extensive course of chemotherapy and radiation therapy. In less than one year the tumor had progressed so that he required feedings through a nasogastric tube. He was cared for at home by his family and the Hospice nursing staff. The author was called when the family began talking about "roots." The patient had developed severe vomiting and the emesis contained a bright yellow substance. The family told the Hospice nurse this might be the "root" they believed had been making him sick. They felt hopeful that he would soon recover. The visiting nurse, startled by these unexpected beliefs, was uncertain how to proceed.

After learning that the patient appeared to be in the terminal phase of his disease, the author proposed that the family might be using traditional beliefs to cope with grief. The family's hope that he would soon recover could represent denial as well as bargaining for more time. It was decided that the nurse would respond to the family in a straightforward fashion and use her skills to provide emotional support. As expected, he died the following day.

While assisting the family with the funeral plans, the nurse learned more about the family's belief in rootwork. The patient had never married and lived with his mother until his death. His brother and sister had moved to the North but returned to North Carolina during the final days of his illness. They reported that the patient had sexual relations with a woman in the community several weeks before he first noticed difficulty swallowing. Returning home, he told his mother he did not trust the woman and thought she might have "put something" in his drink to make him sick. When his swallowing problems persisted, he consulted a herbalist without benefit, and finally sought medical care. When his siblings returned to eastern North Carolina and saw his terminal condition they insisted on taking him first to a palm reader and then to a rootworker. They were instructed to read specific Biblical passages and to administer herbal medicine accompanied by prayers. During one of the Bible readings, the patient vomited the yellow substance, raising hopes that the hex had been removed.

This narrative was shared with the oncologists who had cared for him throughout his long and difficult illness. They remembered him as a pleasant man who, although somewhat distant, took his medications and kept his appointments. They never suspected he believed in rootwork. He was apparently able to simultaneously maintain two seemingly contradictory belief systems about his illness without deleterious impact on his medical care.

Case Seven

Some patients may not be willing to accept medical care when they feel that a root has been worked. The following patient delayed seeking care because of his beliefs until it was too late.

A fifty-year-old black man came to the hospital when the swelling in his legs was so severe that he could no longer walk. In the emergency room he was found to have rectal bleeding along with enlarged lymph glands in his groin, induration of his scrotum and penis, and massive swelling of his legs. The patient was a vague historian and refused to give consent for a needle biopsy of the enlarged glands.

When directly questioned regarding his reasons for refusing further evaluation the patient readily shared his belief that a root had caused his sickness. He reported that the root had been placed by a local bootlegger who was angry because the patient had not paid his bills. The patient witnessed this man "rubbing my chair to dress it before I sat down." Within several days he noticed swelling in his genitals and felt that the hex had taken hold because of sitting on the chair. After two days of treatment in the hospital the leg swelling had decreased enough for the patient to walk and he demanded hospital discharge to seek care from a local rootworker. Two weeks later he returned to the hospital terminally ill. He had been unable to contact his sons whom he had counted on to provide the $400 requested by the rootworker. Feeling that his options were limited, the patient agreed to a lymph node biopsy confirming the diagnosis of metastatic rectal carcinoma. He died several days later.

This case demonstrates that patients may delay seeking care because of beliefs that do not conform with biomedicine. The outcome may be tragic. Health beliefs may also have a significant impact on the utilization of preventive medical services.

Case Eight

Belief in rootwork and hexes is not restricted to the black population. Similar magical practices are occasionally reported by white patients.

An eighty-year-old married white man came to the hospital because of persistent pain in his shoulders and thighs accompanied by severe itching which disturbed his sleep and bedeviled his days. When asked how his symptoms first started, he related the following tale during hospital rounds to an amazed audience of physicians. Five years earlier he had attended a local revival conducted by a charismatic preacher. After an emotional service, all participants were directed to come to the altar to proclaim their faith and receive blessing. The patient, however, stayed in his seat, disapproving of the preacher's "high-minded words and carrying on." After the meeting the preacher walked up to the patient and "fixed me with a terrible stare." Raising his hand dramatically the preacher cast the following hex: "Worms will crawl under your skin—you will be destroyed."

Two weeks later the patient's wife suffered a stroke, confirming his fears that the hex might be real. Her illness made extraordinary demands on this elderly man and he felt that his most important social support was threatened. She did, however, remain in the home.

The patient had an unusual experience the following week. While chopping wood, he noticed that the sunlight appeared unnaturally bright, making everything around him appear magnified. He then saw "creatures or bugs" swarming over his socks and crawling under his pant legs. Frantically, he tried to brush them off but felt that they entered his skin and later traveled throughout his body. His suspicion that the "bugs" were destroying him from the inside was reinforced when he later developed diabetes and thyroid failure. He interpreted his doctor's explanations regarding glandular failure as evidence that "bugs and worms" were, as prophesied, consuming him from within. He also believed the severe itching of his scalp was caused by bugs that came out at night to afflict him. He stayed awake long hours treating his scalp with a variety of salves and ointments to no avail. Other observers, including physicians, were unable after numerous attempts to see these creatures or any evidence of skin disease, but this provided little reassurance and no relief. The patient visited a palmist and a spiritual healer without benefit. He told his physicians about past experiences with rootwork and magic, claiming that his grandfather had nearly died from a hex.

After a muscle biopsy confirmed the diagnosis of eosinophilic fascitis he was begun on low dose prednisone to reduce inflammation in the deep tissues of his upper arms and legs. The patient's itching and other symptoms diminished. However, the medical team thought that relief from the stresses at home might be as important as medication in relieving his suffering. They encouraged the patient to talk about the stresses of caring for a wife with failing health. Directed in this fashion, the patient talked freely of his home problems and mentioned the itching only if asked. Unfortunately, the patient's symptoms promptly recurred when he returned home to his invalid wife despite continuation of his medication. After two years of outpatient treatment, the itching had not improved and he continued to believe it was caused by a hex. His symptoms remitted briefly when his wife was hospitalized for an acute illness only to flare up when she returned home.

Although this man's beliefs differ somewhat from rootwork, his ideas about illness were magical and outside the scope of biotechnical medicine. Animals being introduced into the body by magic is a recurring theme in witchcraft beliefs (Snow 85). His symptoms represented a complex mixture of somatic illness, responses to interpersonal stress, and an idiosyncratic personal belief system. His case also reminds us that we may be unable to relieve a patient's suffering despite our best efforts to provide support and meaning.

These eight cases are a representative rather than an exhaustive catalog of rootwork beliefs in eastern North Carolina. If, as Tinling suggests, patients are asked if they believe "roots" may be involved in their sickness, the number and variety of cases is remarkable (489). In most instances the patient remembers learning about roots from family or friends, frequently during childhood. When sickness strikes, these beliefs are activated, usually in a passing fashion, and the patient wonders if roots might be involved. Most reject the idea and look to the medical doctor for alternative interpretations. If the clinician fails to provide understandable explanations, the patient may return to magical belief systems.

How can clinicians recognize and manage patients who believe they have been hexed? Although no approach works with all cases, the following suggestions have proved useful for the author and colleagues.

The cognitive and cultural gap between physician and patient must first be recognized. The alert clinician listens for clues that the patient's beliefs differ from the biomedical model. Vague or overly dramatic histories, chronic complaints that have not been adequately explained by prior physicians, delay in seeking care, or a sense that the patient is fearful or suspicious that something strange is happening should raise questions about what thoughts and feelings lie behind the patient's behavior. The use of folk descriptions may indicate a traditional illness model. Illness language such as "weak and dizzy," "nerves," "fading," and "poison" are common in eastern North Carolina. Folk beliefs are probably more common, but certainly not restricted to patients from lower socioeconomic and educational groups, blacks and Hispanics, inhabitants of rural areas, and individuals who live at the fringes of society. This author has seen rootwork cases in all ages, although traditional beliefs may be most prevalent in the elderly. Mental illness seems to provide fertile soil for the expression of magical beliefs.

The medical interview is the medium through which the clinician tests and pursues hypotheses about alternate health beliefs and practices. I have found that direct but nonjudgmental questioning is the best way to proceed. Questions such as, "I am wondering if you think roots might be causing your problems?" or "I have seen patients who feel that roots are making them sick. Do you think this could be happening to you?" are generally well accepted. Some patients laugh nervously while others immediately deny such a belief. Quick denial may be a sign of defensiveness. A follow-up question such as, "You seemed pretty quick to say 'No' and I'm wondering if you might feel uncomfortable talking about such things with your doctor?" may convince the patient of the clinician's genuine interest and concern. The reticent patient may share his or her beliefs only when assured of the clinician's willingness to listen.

Not infrequently the patient asks if the doctor believes in roots or has magical powers of his or her own. It is my practice to tell the patient that I have asked about roots because I know other patients who have this belief and have seen how it can complicate medical care if not shared with the doctor. In keeping with my own training in biomedicine, I deny any magical powers, but I reassure the patient that we have successfully treated many patients who believe in hexes. These statements begin the process of sharing and comparing explanatory models.

Kleinman suggests that clinicians elicit an "illness narrative" and develop a "mini-ethnography" and brief life story for each patient (Kleinman 230). Patients can be asked to describe their beliefs and how and from whom they were acquired. Questions such as, "Why do you think you became ill now?" and "What kinds of treatment have you tried and what do you think would be useful now?" can provide new understanding of the illness for both patient and doctor. It cannot be assumed that the patient has a fully articulated explanation of the illness or a consistent set of organized beliefs. In most cases the patient's ideas and feelings are confused and inchoate. By attentively listening to the patient's story, both patient and doctor may discover meanings that neither had expected. The physician gains the opportunity to empathically witness the patient's suffering and establish a healing relationship. The personal, familial, and cultural significance of the symptoms can be pursued and understood.

As the patient's story unfolds, the clinician collects information that can be used to construct the patient's explanatory model of illness. If this model differs significantly from the clinician's, negotiation is needed to develop a model that can be mutually accepted and shared. This task requires flexibility and creativity. If discrepant models are not reconciled, a therapeutic alliance between doctor and patient may be impossible. Negotiation begins with close attention to the patient's language and an appreciation of the patient's daily reality. For example, the doctor can use the patient's feelings of being vulnerable to attack from others as a rationale for building relations with health care providers who will support and shield the patient from harm. A patient's belief in potions or herbal remedies may be honored by the use of vitamin elixirs. Feelings of being out of balance or harmony may be the starting point for informing the patient about the power of medical therapies to restore homeostatic balance and health.

Clinicians should remain mindful that illness threatens the patient with loss of function and that the future may be uncertain. Demoralization is a frequent occurrence for patients who feel socially isolated and stressed and may be particularly severe in patients who believe they are hexed (Snow 83). For the demoralized patient the existence of malevolent forces may not seem fanciful or improbable. Empathic witnessing of the patient's predicament is the starting point for effective management and remoralization. The therapeutic relationship itself may reduce the patient's sense of isolation and helplessness. Other psychotherapeutic interventions include reframing, redirecting, and helping the patient discover practical strategies for approaching life problems. The remoralized patient may still believe in roots but may cope with illness and psychosocial problems in a more adaptive fashion.

When the patient's beliefs produce concerns and conflicts among hospital or clinic staff, a patient care conference may help smooth the waters (Lichstein 128). All involved staff should be included so that information can be shared and consensus reached about a management plan. Similarly, the patient's family should be included in the diagnostic and management process if at all possible. They can provide unique insight about the beliefs of the patient and his or her community. If excluded from the therapeutic network, the family may sabotage the best made plans. On the other hand, a supportive family can be a powerful agent for healthy change.

In summary, the cognitive gap between physician and patient can often be bridged through gentle questioning, nonjudgmental listening, and an attempt to negotiate a shared approach to symptom etiology and management. The clinician is uniquely qualified to develop the flexible, intellectual approach that encompasses the concepts of biotechnical medicine and the cultural perspectives of the individual patient. Although we cannot expect uniform success no matter how skilled and sensitive our approach, dialogue across the technologic-folk interface always improves understanding. With understanding comes the possibility for greater diagnostic accuracy, more appropriate therapy, and greater empathy.

Notes

1. Case One was treated in 1979 at North Carolina Memorial Hospital, Chapel Hill. The remaining cases were treated at the University Medical Center of Eastern Carolina, Pitt County, between 1981 and 1990. All cases were interviewed by the author.

References

Eisenberg, Leon. "What Makes Persons Patients and Patients Well?" *American Journal of Medicine* 69 (1980): 277–86.

———. "The Physician as Interpreter: Ascribing Meaning to the Illness Experience." *Comprehensive Psychiatry* 22 (1981): 239–48.

Engel, George. "The Need for a New Medical Model: A Challenge for Biomedicine." *Science* 196 (1977): 129–36.

Golden, Kenneth M. "Voodoo in Africa and the United States." *American Journal of Psychiatry* 134 (1977): 1,425–27.

Kirkpatrick, Richard A. "Witchcraft and Lupus Erythematosus." *Journal of the American Medical Association* 245 (1981): 1,937.

Kleinman, Arthur. *The Illness Narratives: Suffering, Healing, and the Human Condition.* New York: Basic, 1988.

Kleinman, Arthur, Leon Eisenberg, and Byron Good. "Culture, Illness, and Care: Clinical Lessons from Anthropologic and Cross-Cultural Research." *Annals of Internal Medicine* 88 (1978): 251–58.

Leininger, Madeleine. "Witchcraft Practices and Psychocultural Therapy with Urban U.S. Families." *Human Organization* 32 (1973): 73–83.

Lichstein, Peter R. "Can a Physician Heal a Hex?" *Hospital Practice* (1982): 125–32.

Lyles, Michael R., and James R. Hillard. "Root Work and the Refusal of Surgery." *Psychosomatics* 23 (1982): 663.

Mack, Ronald. "Through All Thy Veins Shall Run a Cold and Drowsy Humor: Nightshade Poisoning." *North Carolina Medical Journal* 48 (1987): 258–59.

Snow, Loudell. "Folk Medical Beliefs and Their Implications for Care of Patients." *Annals of Internal Medicine* 81 (1974): 82–96.

Spanos, Nicholas P. "Witchcraft in Histories of Psychiatry: A Critical Analysis and an Alternative Conceptualization." *Psychological Bulletin* 85 (1978): 417.

Tinling, David C. "Voodoo, Root Work, and Medicine." *Psychosomatic Medicine* 29 (1967): 483–90.

Weimer, Sanford R., and Norbett L. Mintz. "Health Practice at the Technologic/Folk Interface: Witchcraft as a Culture-Specific Diagnosis." *International Journal of Psychiatric Medicine* 7 (1977): 351–62.

Zola, I. K. "Studying the Decision to See the Doctor." *Advances in Psychosomatic Medicine* 8 (1972): 216–36.

7. The Cultural Epidemiology of Spiritual Heart Trouble

Linda A. Camino

During an eighteen-month period in 1983 and 1984, I undertook field research to investigate health and illness beliefs and practices in an African-American neighborhood, which I have called Prosperity Heights. Prosperity Heights is located in a large piedmont city in Virginia.

Though most of the discourse about health and illness among neighborhood residents is replete with a wide range of ethnomedical disorders such as "arthritis of the eyeball," "high blood," "low blood," or "nerves," one of the most compelling is an illness called spiritual heart trouble. Spiritual heart trouble warranted detailed consideration for several reasons: many of its associated symptoms exhibit a pattern of somatic distress that is also often expressed in depressive disorders; other symptoms reflect behavior and/or mood disruptions, suggesting that the illness is overlaid with a fan of personal, social, and cultural meanings; and finally, the prevalence of spiritual heart trouble appeared rather high, although it has never been formally reported in the research literature.

Spiritual heart trouble is experienced by not just anyone in Prosperity Heights, but rather by those individuals belonging to a local Pentecostal Holiness Church. Several months into the research and continuing until I left Prosperity Heights, I began to attend Sunday morning service at Holiness Church, one of three churches located in the neighborhood. I knew from the work of other researchers that religious services frequently provide fruitful material for studies of health and illness. What I was unprepared for, however, is the overwhelming extent to which health-related issues permeate this particular church. Sermons are thick with references to sickness as one of the primary wages of sin, and to well-being as the result of leading a life that is "lined up with God."

Members of the congregation who are ailing and unable to attend services are routinely announced and prayers offered for them. Revivals and prayer meetings occur frequently, and people with all manner of problems move through a prayer line to receive blessings and laying-on-of-hands healing from the pastor or another minister as an established part of the Sunday service.

Spiritual heart trouble is mentioned specifically by the pastor in sermons and is named by individuals in their interactions with ministers while in the prayer line. As will be discussed in this chapter, spiritual heart trouble begins when people allow Satan or demons to be received into their hearts. Forces of evil are thought to overpower and replace the spiritually good forces of holiness, grace, joy, and desire. In Holiness Church the heart is construed as a locus for human spirituality in addition to the center of the body's circulatory system. This chapter aims to present a clear articulation of the distress that spiritual heart trouble imparts through a detailed analysis of the symbolic references attached to the heart and blood in the religious belief system.

Holiness Church has a formal membership of approximately 175 persons, but attendance at Sunday morning service averages 120. The data reported here were obtained primarily through participant observation and semistructured interviews with an opportunistic sampling of 20 persons who appeared in the prayer line on account of spiritual heart trouble and who agreed to be interviewed. The interview schedule consisted of three sections: a demographic profile; a series of open-ended questions designed to elicit indigenous explanatory models of illness, based on the work of Kleinman and others; and a check list concerning the manifestation of autonomic nervous system symptoms in relation to emotional distress (Lex). Each interview lasted between two and three hours. In addition, informal interviews were conducted with the pastor.

Profile of Spiritual Heart Trouble

Spiritual heart trouble afflicts those persons who are predominantly from a rural background and who have converted to, not been ascribed by birth, membership in the Pentecostal Holiness faith. More than twice as many women (fourteen) as men (six) reported the illness and the parameters on which they varied are age and marital status: whereas females ranged from sixteen to sixty-three years of age and all but one were married or divorced, all men except one were in their twenties and single.

Spiritual heart trouble exhibits a range of symptoms: "heavy heart,"

"heart beating fast," uncontrollable drowsiness, interrupted sleep, headaches, weakness, dizziness, "sayings things I shouldn't," and "loss of spiritual joy or desire." No one remembered a precise point in time to which they could attribute its onset. Spiritual heart trouble was assessed as "real bad" by everyone in its severity and the greatest fear held by all was that, if untreated, it would lead to spiritual death (which was "just as good as real dead"). In addition to the therapy people sought from the church ministers, everyone employed self-treatment modalities, including taking aspirin, fasting, reading Bible passages, and praying. It is considered that anyone may contract spiritual heart trouble and that its genesis is situational; only two persons claimed that heredity played a part in the appearance of the illness ("coming down through the family"). In striking contrast to the trend to seek help for the problem from a Pentecostal minister, only one person also brought her complaint to an orthodox physician, and only when the physical pain grew unbearable for her (the medical diagnosis was ulcers).

Although sufferers were unable to pinpoint a time for the onset of spiritual heart trouble, they were decisive concerning explicit circumstances which they viewed as the major contributing factors for its appearance. These circumstances assign responsibility to persons connected to the patients, such as spouses, children, parents (consanguineal relatives were named most often), fellow employees, work supervisors, and regular service personnel.

In sum, spiritual heart trouble is suffered by members of the Pentecostal Holiness faith who preponderantly come from a rural background and who are predominantly women. Of the range of symptoms listed above, the three regarded as most important and reported by every individual are "heavy heart," "saying things I shouldn't," and "loss of spiritual joy or desire." Those who suffer spiritual heart trouble consider it to be a serious illness whose debilitating effects impinge upon the routines of their lives and which, if unchecked, can lead to spiritual death. Every patient named another person connected to him or her when asked: "Why do you think it started when it did?" "Was there anything different that happened in your life at that time?"

The foregoing represents an overview of spiritual heart trouble, showing its structural aspects. It is worthwhile to review individual case histories, for these demonstrate how the processes of the illness operate in actual practice, and how, in a given situation, an individual manifests distress in the idiom of this ethnomedical illness.

Case Examples

Rebecca T. is a forty-seven-year-old woman with three daughters, two of whom (ages seventeen and fourteen) live at home. Mrs. T. is divorced and works in the medical section (although she is a licensed practical nurse) of the private hospital located near Prosperity Heights. Mrs. T. was brought up as a Baptist but was rebaptized or "saved" in the Pentecostal Holiness faith approximately five years ago. Her conversion represented a major turning point in her life because she reports her boyfriend and her father, who have provided her with some financial support, both left her on account of her new convictions. "Then I really knew what it was to be alone in your faith," she states. For several Sundays she appeared in the prayer line at church because of "weakness, sadness, worry, no joy, yelling at the kids, and a heavy heart," which she experienced "all the time" and which caused her "not to want to do anything." Mrs. T. laments the fact that she is not "growing spiritually." She sees the cause of her spiritual heart trouble as worry and responsibility over her youngest daughter who was a formerly obedient and respectful child, but who recently began to play hooky from school and was picked up by the police on several minor charges. Mrs. T. asserts that though she herself had led a problem-filled life, she had always taken pride in her ability to "look out" for herself. In contrast, worry about her children, particularly the youngest, had sapped her emotional strength for some time. Mrs. T. believes that her worry constitutes a sin and that it is contributing to her spiritual death.

Another case involves Pearl C., age forty, who lives with her husband, mother, and youngest daughter. Mrs. C.'s problems, too, manifested themselves in a "heavy heart," "saying things I shouldn't," "no more spiritual joy," an overwhelming desire to stay in bed throughout the day, and debilitating stomach pains. These last have compelled her to regularly attend the gastroenteritis clinic at the university hospital for the past several years, where they have been diagnosed as ulcers. Mrs. C. contends her problems arise out of an inherited tendency to worry and the difficult conditions of her family life. She reports that throughout her married life her husband has beaten her, that she had managed to endure this, but that other recent pressing problems combined to lower her ability to cope. These were the pregnancy of her thirteen-year-old daughter, her mother's terminal cancer, and her husband's serious injury which he sustained in an automobile accident (he had been the main financial provider for the family). Mrs. C. feels exceedingly guilty over the fact that she finds it difficult to support her relatives emotionally or financially in their particular crises since she herself has trouble, and she laments the fact that no one is caring for her. This in itself produces another form of guilt, for she worries all the more that she has doubted God, who is supposed to be her savior; hence she has sinned and fears that she may die spiritually.

Paul W. is twenty-nine, single, works on the janitorial staff at the nearby university, and shares an apartment with another single man. In addition to the core symptoms of spiritual heart trouble, he reports headaches, inability to sleep at night, and feeling sluggish during the day. His distress began when the "higher ups" moved him to another building to work where he encountered a fellow employee who was the nephew of the man who had helped Mr. W. secure his job. The employee tried to manipulate Mr. W. into doing his work. At first the coworker drew Mr. W.'s sympathy and he helped the man, but he then became indignant over the injustice displayed by the supervisor, who told Mr. W. that he was working too slowly and warned that he could easily be fired because plenty of other people would like to have the job. Mr. W. wanted to inform the supervisor that he was actually helping another worker, but was coldly told by the coworker himself that he could also get fired easily on these grounds. Mr. W. was placed in a perfect double bind: his religious morals and indirect social debt to his coworker prompted his assistance, but his job performance appeared less than satisfactory as a result. This led to anxiety about losing his job and feelings of guilt and indecisiveness about confronting the coworker directly. Mr. W. is at a loss as to what to do and notes that God is no longer "touching" him.

These examples vividly illustrate the circumstances of spiritual heart trouble patients that lie behind the formal profile. The most noteworthy aspects of the precipitating events that give rise to spiritual heart trouble are role confusion and conflict over priorities. Mrs. T. was anguished over her inability to control her adolescent daughter and was caught up in trying to assess what her job as a mother is. Mrs. C. was required to give emotional support and attention simultaneously as a wife, mother, and daughter to members of her family who suffered problems at the same time that she herself was ill. Paul W. wanted to keep his job and live up to the moral standards of Christian charity while he endured the manipulation of his coworker and the strain of carrying out the jobs of two people.

Analysis

A review of the reported symptoms reveals that a pattern of somatic as well as behavior distress is exhibited in spiritual heart trouble: accelerated heart beat, "heavy heart," drowsiness, interrupted sleep, headaches, weakness, dizziness, "loss of joy or desire," and "saying things I shouldn't." If the physical symptoms were to be isolated from the behavioral ones and tested, it might be found that they signify the presence of underlying organic disease. Such diagnostic tests were not performed in this study, and thus it cannot be positively ruled out that the symptoms reflect serious organic disease.

Nevertheless, one of the most elementary observations that can be made about the physical symptoms is that they are vague and, as such, closely resemble those characteristic of a process known in orthodox medicine as somatization, defined as: "The articulation of emotional problems and psychosocial stress by way of physical symptomatology. . . . Patients who somatize either have no organic disease and recurrently present with physical complaints or have verifiable organic problems, but amplify their symptoms" (Rosen et al. 493).

Several researchers note that the tendency to somatize appears frequently in undereducated and working-class patients, or in those who belong to various subcultural and religious groups (Kleinman). Indeed, somatization is regarded as an idiomatic way of expressing emotional distress in groups who either lack an orthodox psychological vocabulary or among whom mental affliction is stigmatized.

If the vague somatic symptoms of spiritual heart trouble can be seen as evidence of somatization processes, this would point to the hypothesis that the illness is a psychosomatic one. Closer inspection of other features of spiritual heart trouble also supports this view. First, there is a group of complaints, which, although they do not express dysphoria in elaborated psychological terms, nonetheless allude to it: "loss of joy or desire," "heavy heart," and "saying things I shouldn't." Second, the very assertions in the patients' own explanatory models that worry is both cause and result of spiritual heart trouble appear to demonstrate an indigenous perception of significant psychological involvement.

But to draw such a conclusion and leave the matter at that is to leave unanswered many remaining and pressing epidemiological questions. Why does the illness occur among Pentecostals? Why is its cause most often imputed to be a problematic relationship with a consanguineal relative? Because "loss of joy or desire," a "heavy or funny heart," and "saying things I shouldn't" were the symptoms that were consistently reported by every patient, it may be assumed that they carry great significance in the articulation of the illness. What are the meanings attached to them? And finally, why is it the heart and not some other body part that is singled out as the locus of "dis-ease" in this community?

These questions can only be answered if the various features of spiritual heart trouble are examined against the sociocultural context in which it occurs. To this end, the structure of Pentecostal belief, specifically the system of the Pentecostal Holiness Church, will be explored. It should be borne in mind that although this analysis shifts to one that primarily employs anthropological concepts, these considerably overlap with those used in medical and psychological studies as well.

Spiritual Heart Trouble in Anthropological Perspective

Pentecostalism represents a fundamentalist religious sect, claiming a black membership as high as four million in contemporary America (Richardson and Wright 51), the majority of which cluster at the low end of the socioeconomic pole. These "spirit-filled churches" practice evangelical preaching, a "born again" relationship with God, and place a premium on living along guidelines promulgated in the Bible that are literally interpreted. The services are characterized by emotional, at times passionate, expression, and membership entails a comprehensive commitment on the part of the individual for most churches not only offer Sunday service, but also expect attendance at Sunday School classes, weeknight prayer meetings, morning and afternoon Sunday services, revivals, and other activities. Pentecostal congregations are well aware that their belief in demonic or divine possession, casting out of demons, laying on of hands, and speaking in tongues often are regarded by outsiders as curious or freakish.

This summary of general aspects of Pentecostalism characterizes the congregation of Holiness Church in Prosperity Heights. The immediate effect of these features is to bestow a sense of differentiation among the faithful vis-à-vis secular society and even against other African-American groups, with a concomitant enhancement of a sense of solidarity among the church members. The moral boundary between the congregation and the rest of secular humanity is well demarcated and assumes several expressions. In the parlance of their religious conviction, for example, members of Holiness Church refer to themselves as "saints" or "saved," while outsiders are designated "sinners" or "unsaved." Similarly, the physical boundaries for the church are well demarcated: the doors are usually kept closed during any kind of service and they are regularly anointed with blessed olive oil to ward off evil influences.

Yet, within the bounds of the moral collective, the boundaries are more informal, displaying a type of organization which Victor Turner refers to in *The Ritual Process* as communitas. The social and cultural arrangements of communitas stand in direct opposition to the formal, well-defined and insulated role structure that characterizes mainstream society; communitas organization emphasizes loosely drawn divisions and classifications, and highlights intimacy and egalitarianism. Moreover, Turner argues in *Dramas, Fields, and Metaphors* that groups that are socially marginal or "structurally inferior" within mainstream society are especially prone to organize themselves along the lines of communitas and will fashion their interactions in fairly standardized forms: the assumption that mystical rather than practical bonds unite the members, the massive application of fictive sibling relationships, and the dictate that material property should be shunned. Following Turner's formulations, the members of Holiness Church represent such a group on three accounts: they are members of a racial minority, they are members of an ideological minority, and they live, for the most part, lives that are materially meager. Furthermore, the members assert that they are related to one another through Christ, that they are all equal "in the eyes of God"; all routinely refer to one another as "brother or sister" with the exception of the clergy, who are called "elder" or "minister"; and people liberally contribute to the church fund as many as three times per service.

Given the portrayal of Holiness Church as organized around the principle of communitas, it is apparent that the sense of solidarity that is thus created is focused, on the one hand, on a notion of external uniqueness and separation and, on the other hand, on an internal feeling of equality, cooperation, and fellowship.

What is the major implication of communitas for the identity of the individual within Holiness Church? It is one that is held to have internal and external features. The opposition between an inner and outer identity finds expression in all types of services where a great deal of sermonistic rhetoric is devoted to "being really you" as opposed to being the person who enacts roles in secular life. The religious identity is held to be the "true" one and "real" in character. But all members must possess this identity, making it one that is shared, not singular.

If we compare such a notion of identity with that operating in middle-class white America, we find a significant difference. In this sphere, there is a similar principle between inner and outer identities, yet there is a conviction that the inner identity is regarded as particularistic or idiosyncratic, not communal, creating a sentiment in which all believe themselves and are believed by others to be entirely different from everyone else. In the secular mainstream United States most people feel they have an internal component that is private and, hence, one that no one else can see. This view is related to the understanding that people are able to personalize their roles and status; that is, while the behavior of an individual enacting a role will reflect institutionalized features, it will also reflect the private personality enacting the role. *Within* the structure of Holiness Church no one has to personalize his or her role because they are all relatively the same. It is not that Pentecostal ideology completely strips away personalism or idiosyncrasy, for each individual is held to be special to God, who has given him or her unique talents, but these talents or abilities are not supposed to be used as the means to achieve personal ends. Instead, they are to be directed toward the moral collective composed of fellow Pentecostals and God. The inner identity of the individual in Holiness Church is thus transparent, not hidden as in the secular mainstream United States: it is one that God, or Satan, or a fellow Pentecostal can "see."

Such a construction of identity bears directly upon the notion of selfhood. Whereas white middle-class Americans regard the self as built around the "ego," a point of stability or reference separating the inner and outer selves, the Pentecostal self is presumed to be fluid because it derives from the fluctuating presence of good or evil within the person. In order to clarify this point, it is useful to consider Pentecostal cosmology.

In Pentecostal belief the universe is divided into the secular world of humankind and the other world, which is again sectioned into God's kingdom, shared also by angels and saved souls, and Hell, where the Devil, his demons, and damned souls dwell. Humankind comes into the world with a potential of joining Satan's ranks, for people are born with original sin. They have, however, the opportunity to achieve redemption if they repent of their sins, accept Jesus Christ as their personal savior, and live in careful accordance with guidelines promulgated in the Bible.

While this can be an easy task to perform, the true hardship is continual resistance to Satan and his demons who are wily, crafty, persistent, and ruthless in their attempts to capture souls for their ranks. It is held, furthermore, that demons not only are motivated in their machinations by their instruction to seize souls for Satan, but also because of their drive to maintain existence; that is, demons must dwell in a concrete place in addition to the abstract territory of Hell, and they find humans a comfortable and agreeable habitat. When a demon (and it is pictured as a small ugly monkey, perhaps to signify its humanoid, but not human qualities) permeates a human being, it attacks the mind or body first, and then goes to work on the spirit. Demons "poison" people, and any imperfection of behavior or any sickness is considered to be the result of a demon invasion. But just as demons can penetrate a human being, fill him or her with evil and corruption, and cause organic, mental, or spiritual debilitation, so can the Holy Ghost enter or "touch" a person, filling him or her with divine grace, and therefore give health.

This means that the self as a locus of responsibility is one that is capable of being shifted. When an individual in Holiness Church exhibits sickness, people say that he or she has sinned by allowing a demon to enter his or her being. Yet, once this occurs, the responsibility is transferred to Satan, and the individual is consequently regarded as seriously debilitated in the ability to help himself or herself. The obverse, of course, holds as well: an individual is accountable for his or her health, yet the healthy state is ultimately attributed to the bestowal of God's grace. Thus, to exist in a state of health or of illness the individual must give over a part of the self and the remittance is expressed in metaphors of death. When an individual experiences possession of the Holy Ghost during regular church service, people call it "slaying for the Lord," and indeed they can enact it in the extreme through trance behavior. Again, when a person becomes "possessed of" or "oppressed by" a demon which brings forth illness, a part of the spiritual self is said to die. What dies is the self joined with God and which is now filled with evil; similarly in "slaying for the Lord," just the amount of evil intrusion must be made to die before it can be refilled with God's grace in order to live again in health.

Thus far, it has been established that the organization of Holiness Church is built upon the foundation of loose internal boundaries and a well-drawn boundary between itself and the secular community. The internal-external theme, moreover, extends to the conception of the individual himself or herself within the religious community. Pentecostalism assumes that a secular identity is superfluous, while the religious one is real and one that is shared, not separated, from other members. The way in which selfhood is construed posits a tenuous and permeable boundary between the self and God, self and Satan, and the self and other selves.

According to Mary Douglas (136–52), groups which possess clear external boundaries and blurred, confused internal demarcations, will not only exhibit extensive internal-external motifs, but will posit also that the problem of evil or misfortune arises from within the ranks. Here, where internal boundaries are nebulous, a confusion of roles exists; they are amorphous, contradictory, or confused to the point where they become impossible for individuals to perform. Douglas further hypothesizes that such organizational features go hand in hand with witchcraft or dualistic religious cosmologies, where the witch or the Devil personifies evil, acting against the fundamental purity of the social as well as the individual bodies.

If the cases of the people with spiritual heart trouble are recalled, one of the salient features of the accounts of precipitating causes is indeed confusion of roles and/or moral categories. Mrs. T. viewed her problems as resulting from the moral conflict between her religious convictions and the absence of these in her father and boyfriend, the contradiction between her ability to "look out for herself" and her responsibility toward a daughter whom she could no longer control, and the opposition between her inclination to worry about her child and the guilt which emanated from such feelings due to the fact that worry constitutes a sin. Similarly, Pearl C. felt conflict about her inability to give emotional support to her thirteen-year-old daughter and her terminally ill mother while she herself was ill, and about her financial and moral need to remain with a husband who beat her (divorce in Holiness Church is considered a sin). Mrs. C. worried, moreover, about her worry and felt guilty for doubting God. And so it is with all the cases: each patient had strands of conflicting and competing obligations which they found impossible to order with priorities. The ambiguity produced frustrations, as Douglas predicts.

But the conflicting and ambiguous roles of these patients do not spring merely from the loose organization within Holiness Church, but from confusions in the secular world as well. Why should such ambiguity give rise to illness if, after all, blurred boundaries between self and other, according to Pentecostal doctrine, are considered normal and even healthy? Moreover, patients attributed the genesis of spiritual heart trouble not entirely to the Devil and his demons, nor indeed to a fellow member of the church, but, in fact, to people who are closely related to the patient by virtue of social circumstance in the secular world.

On the basis of these observations, it is possible to hypothesize that it is the dissonance between an individual's socialization to a role prescribed

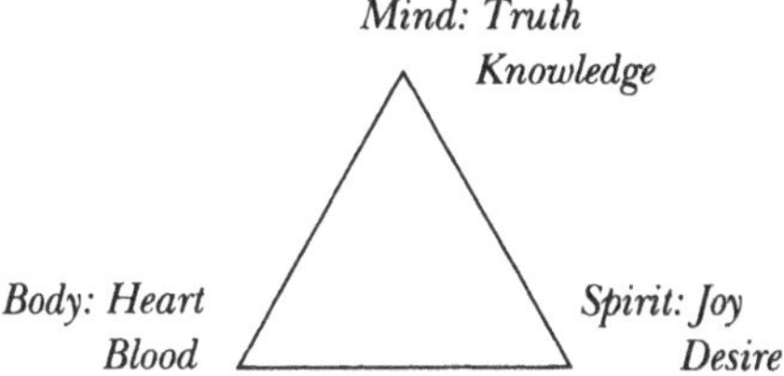

Figure 7.1 Model of Health in Holiness Church

by Pentecostal doctrine and that which is dictated by the constraints and configurations of his or her secular life that constitutes the basic operative cause of spiritual heart trouble. To examine this hypothesis, this analysis must be pushed beyond a cursory look at Pentecostal cosmological structure toward an inspection of the core affective and behavioral symptoms presented by each patient: "heavy heart," "loss of joy or desire," and "saying things I shouldn't." As will be demonstrated, these symptoms carry a rich array of symbolic messages that make clearer the import of emotional, cultural, and social factors in the pathogenesis of the affliction.

The Core Symptoms of Spiritual Heart Trouble: Cognition and Affect

The members of Holiness Church posit that human essence is composed of three irreducible elements: body, mind, and spirit. The elements form a tripartite foundation of ideal existence, and a harmonious relationship must exist between all three in order to achieve a state of health. The focus of the body is on the heart and blood, that of the mind on truth and knowledge, and that of the spirit on joy and desire for God (see figure 7.1).

To begin to decode these constructions, it is useful to follow Victor Turner's recommendations to review the indigenous exegeses themselves (*The Forest of Symbols* 49). The following texts represent the range of explanations that I collected.

Body: The heart is:

1. an organ that pumps blood
2. what carries the perpetuation of life; it is the issue of your life
3. what you use to love other people
4. what you should put into your work (enthusiasm)
5. what breaks if you are too sad

6. what bursts if you have joy
7. what comes out of you if you have problems
8. what loves God
9. how you know God
10. what speaks to God
11. what knows the truth
12. what God is in the church
13. where the Holy Ghost dwells
14. what demons eat
15. where Satan plants his evil seeds

Body: Blood is:

1. the stuff that runs in veins—what the heart pumps
2. what women issue in monthlies
3. the thing that connects us
4. a relationship
5. what we are born in
6. what carries our sins through the human race
7. the guilt of murder—having someone's blood on your hand
8. what the animals in the Bible died in
9. what God died in so we can live
10. the blood of Jesus; it protects us from demons
11. the thing that relates man to God

Mind: Knowledge is:

1. experience—what your mind stores—what the heart stores
2. sexual intercourse in the language of the Bible
3. what Adam and Eve ate
4. God's way—saying it right
5. how you know right from wrong
6. what causes you to worry

Mind: Truth is:

1. the right way to live
2. what God teaches
3. what gives you everlasting life
4. healing; when someone knows the truth he is healed

Spirit: Joy is:

1. the wish to be with a man or woman
2. the feeling of being alive

3. the feeling of loving other people
4. what happens when God touches your heart
5. what dies when Satan gets in your mind and heart

Spirit: Desire is:

1. what makes you want to be with a man or woman
2. what makes you want to be with people you love
3. what brings you to God
4. what you lose in spiritual heart trouble

Moving beyond the indigenous exegeses, which at first sight appear to be a random collection of references, we find that several recurrent themes are disclosed. Turner shows that three properties are contained in dominant symbols: condensation, unification of disparate significata, and polarization of meaning (*The Forest of Symbols* 28). Each of these is evidenced here. With respect to condensation, the span of references for the heart, knowledge, truth, joy, and desire describe them as well as the institution of Pentecostalism itself. For example, the heart denotes a physiological organ; it states a relationship between people; and it binds humankind and God as well. The heart as God is metaphorical of his vital place in the religious body. Blood signifies the organic processes of circulation, menstruation, birth, or death; it portrays mother-child bonds, the interrelationship of humanity, or the disruption of relationships (murder); and on another level represents the spiritual body of individuals interlinked through Pentecostalism (the blood of Jesus protects the congregation from demons). Each of the remaining components demonstrates similar symbolic associations. Here we have evidence which supports Douglas's hypothesis that the structure and function of the human body is perceived as consonant with the social and ideological structures and functions; that is, the physical, social, and ideological bodies are declared to be homologous: each is conceived of in terms of the others using the same elements, so that the diagram might be amended as shown in figure 7.2.

It follows that just as the parts of the individual must interconnect and operate in harmony to maintain health, so must those component elements of the social and ideological bodies; and indeed, it is necessary for all of the systems to engage and work in triadic unity.

The second major feature of the textual referents for the heart, blood, knowledge, joy, and desire is that they clearly articulate ambivalence, simultaneously encoding contradictory qualities. Accordingly, the

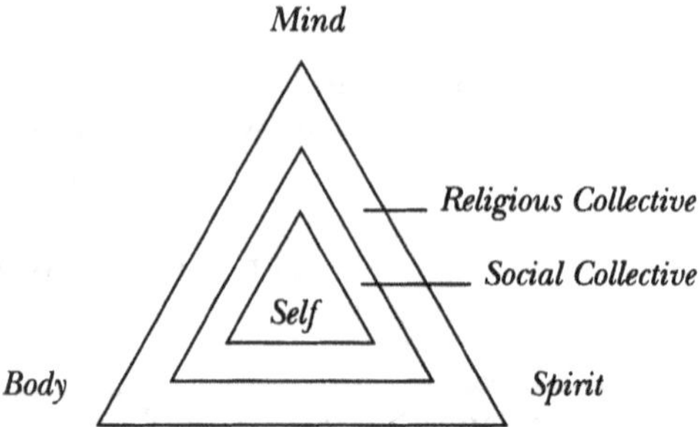

Figure 7.2 Model of the Self, Social and Religious Collectives

heart embodies joy as well as sadness, and is the dwelling place of the Holy Ghost in addition to what demons eat or where Satan sows evil; blood signifies both life and death, protection and violence; knowledge indicates right and wrong; joy expresses life and death; and desire signifies motivation or apathy. The exception to the trend is truth, which carries consistent meanings as a correct way of living, God's teachings, everlasting life, and healing. Truth has important bearings on the treatment for spiritual heart trouble (Camino 1986).

The third aspect of the span of referents for the heart, blood, knowledge, joy, and desire is the unification of polarized semantic terms. Turner describes this feature as follows. "At one pole cluster a set of referents to grossly physiological character, relating general human experience of an emotional kind. At the other pole cluster a set of referents to moral norms and principles governing the social structure" (Turner *The Forest of Symbols*, 53). The inventory of such polarized meanings in Holiness Church is summarized in table 7.1.

It is evident that the three properties of dominant symbols—condensation, unification of disparate significata, and polarization of meaning—derive their power from the various aggregations of references they can employ. They are, Turner tells us, "multivocal"; and their mixture of references embodies a tension-like energy, capable of affecting potent forces in social interaction. We have seen that, in the conceptualization of members of Holiness Church, the body as heart and blood, the mind as knowledge, and the spirit as joy and desire symbolize the configurations of the individual, social, and ideological bodies; they embrace the contradictions inherent in these configurations; and they articulate the physical and emotional as surely as the normative and cognitive aspects of human experience. This last feature becomes especially salient in the consider-

Table 7.1 Polarized Meanings of Dominant Symbols in Holiness Church

	Orectic, Affective	Normative, Cognitive
Heart	1. Love 2. Joy 3. Sadness 4. Enthusiasm 5. Cannibalism ("what demons eat")	1. Continuity of Mankind 2. Unity of Pentecostalism
Blood	1. Menstruation 2. Birth 3. Death 4. Violence 5. Nurture	1. Unity of human and animal life 2. Mankind 3. Union of mankind and God in God and Pentecostalism
Knowledge	1. Sexual intercourse 2. Danger, evil 3. Worry	1. Morality 2. Pentecostalism
Joy	1. Sexual attraction 2. Love	1. Morality 2. Pentecostalism
Desire	1. Sexual attraction	1. Social unions 2. Union of mankind and God
Summary	Emotions themselves or experiences charged with heightened sentiments	Continuity and unity in social and ideological spheres

ation of ethnomedical illness, for it is within this domain that culture influences universal psychobiological effects and molds them into culturally recognized or culture-specific disorders.

Given this consideration, it becomes clear why the heart in Holiness Church is chosen as the representative locus of distress. If the texts of the references for body, mind, and spirit components are examined further, it is evident that it is the heart that consistently crosses all the classifications, mixing and reformulating all other metaphors to create a myriad of meanings. When the heart is paired with blood, it is the thing that pumps and circulates both a physiological substance and a metaphysical substance bringing people and spirits together; when linked with knowledge, it is a storage and exchange center for all that represents experience; when associated with joy and desire, it interconnects humans with God. The heart can love other people, motivate actions, produce emotions, talk to God, know the truth, receive God or Satan, become the food of demons, and even become the incarnation of God within the church. Because the heart binds the elements of the entire symbolic system together, because it converts and reformulates them, and because it transcends them, the heart is the vital center of the semantic networks of body, mind, and spirit, and indeed of the moral universe in Holiness Church.

What, then, do the symptoms "heavy heart," "saying things I shouldn't," and "loss of joy or desire" signify? Fundamentally, they represent the reverse patterns of a healthy person's experience, which is a light heart, speaking from the heart, and the possession of joy or desire. But through their metaphorical associations, clustering around conceptions of body, mind, and spirit, they declare a rupture of the person from the social and ideological systems and depict a process that is perceived as the departure of the self from the unity and harmony considered to be good health. For example, since the heart "loves other people," "loves God," and "knows the truth," a "heavy heart" symbolizes a disturbance in these chains of relationships—relationships which people must have if they are to exist in physical, emotional, and spiritual health. Because saying it right—"in God's way"—betokens health of the mind, "saying things I shouldn't" signifies a separation between the individual and God. And because joy and desire properly connect people ("the feeling of loving other people") as well as people and God ("what happens when God touches your heart" or "what brings you to God"), "loss of joy or desire" similarly symbolizes a rupture in emotional, social, and spiritual relationships. These ruptures, breaks, and separations, in effect, serve to construct a boundary between the ailing individual and his or her social and religious connections. They announce that the sick person is alone, cut off from others—antithetical to the healthy self, a self that must be a relational or shared self with permeable boundaries.

Thus it is that all the patients with spiritual heart trouble spoke at length about the importance of interpersonal conflict in the etiology of their illness, the worry about God no longer "touching" them, and the feeling of "wanting to be alone," "not wanting to go out," "not wanting to get up in the morning," "not wanting to see other people," and "not wanting to know God" as consequences of their illness. Spiritual heart troubled patients are rendered socially and spiritually isolated.

Conclusion

What does all this symbolism have to do with the illness spiritual heart trouble? Most essentially, it enables us to locate spiritual heart trouble within indigenous idioms to tell us what it is, and where, when, and how it occurs. Although it may seem patently obvious to clinicians that the illness may be a label for underlying anxiety or depressive disorder induced by reaction of the autonomic nervous system, it is noteworthy that a core triad of symptoms—"heavy heart," "saying things I shouldn't," and "loss of joy or desire" were the locus of distress for every patient. Do particular illness symptoms always have a "meaning" beyond that of signaling general responses to stressful stimuli?

In this anthropological investigation of the symptomatic meanings of spiritual heart trouble there has been no attempt made to correlate symptomatic expression with the personalities of the patients, though it is not unlikely the illness has a component of psychosomatic pathology. Above all, it is clear that a striking resemblance exists between the precipitating events in each case history—events that apply to the meanings of the core triad of symptoms, which themselves attach to vital Pentecostal principles. In this way, the idiom of spiritual heart trouble represents not only psychosomatic, but sociosomatic (Lipowski) distress as well.

Spiritual heart trouble is experienced by low-income black Pentecostals who form a disenfranchised and marginal group in the United States. The symptoms "heavy heart," "saying things I shouldn't," and "loss of joy or desire" communicate essential conceptions of body, mind, and spirit and, by extension, of the place and purpose of the individual within the moral collective of the church. An episode of spiritual heart trouble tells of the clash between these moral imperatives and actual secular life. It heightens and makes evident the themes of "insiders" and "outsiders" and consequent boundaries that underpin much of Pentecostal belief.

Thus far we have been concerned with establishing a frame of reference for spiritual heart trouble to articulate its relationship with sociocultural and psychological events. Although this chapter is based on field rather than clinical research, there are several practical considerations pertaining to spiritual heart trouble that clinicians can profitably employ.

Most essentially, clinicians should be alerted to a possible relationship between the ethnomedical illness spiritual heart trouble and anxiety and depressive disorders. Patients may not present directly a complaint of "spiritual heart trouble," but may cast their problems as "loss of joy or desire," "saying things I shouldn't," or "funny or heavy heart." References to disturbances in the heart may be especially amplified by patients, because many low-income African-American patients learn to present their distress with somatic valences in medical facilities (Camino 1989).

Because spiritual heart trouble contributes to lowered self-esteem and feelings of isolation, clinicians are well advised to take an active approach in interviews by volunteering questions such as "Do you suffer from loss of joy or desire? Heavy heart?" "Some patients suffer from spiritual heart trouble. Could that be your problem?" Especially in light of the several other vague somatic symptoms that attend spiritual heart trouble, such as headaches and dizziness, these questions can help focus initial interviews and thereby save extraneous medical workups. Of course, stereotyping patients according to their ethnicity or race is a dangerous enterprise and can severely compromise a beneficial practitioner-patient relationship as well as the delivery of appropriate services. Therefore, it should be stressed that any such probes used by a clinician be phrased in an open-ended and nonjudgmental manner.

References

Camino, Linda A. "Ethnomedical Illnesses and Nonorthodox Healing Practices in a Black Neighborhood in the American South: How They Work and What They Mean." Dissertation. University of Virginia, 1986.

———. "Nerves, Worriation, and Black Women: A Community Study in the American South." *Gender, Health and Illness: The Case of Nerves*. Ed. Dona L. Davis and Setha Low. New York: Hemisphere, 1989. 295–314.

Douglas, Mary. *Natural Symbols*. New York: Vintage, 1973.

Kleinman, Arthur. *Patients and Healers in the Context of Culture: An Exploration of the Borderline between Anthropology, Medicine, and Psychiatry*. Berkeley: University of California Press, 1980.

Kleinman, Arthur, Leon Eisenberg, and Byron Good. "Culture, Illness, and Care: Clinical Lessons from Anthropological and Cross-Cultural Research." *Annals of Internal Medicine* 88 (1978): 251–88.

Lex, Barbara. "Voodoo Death: New Thoughts on an Old Explanation." *American Anthropologist* 76 (1974): 818–23.

Lipowski, Z. J. "Psychosomatic Medicine in a Changing Society: Some Current Trends in Theory and Research." *Comprehensive Psychiatry* 14 (1977): 203–15.

Richardson, Harry V., and Nathan Wright, Jr. "Afro-American Religion." *The Black American Reference Book*. Ed. Mable Smythe. Englewood Cliffs, N.J.: Prentice-Hall, 1976. 492–514.

Rosen, Gary, Arthur Kleinman, and Wayne Katon. "Somatization in Family Practice: A Biopsychosocial Approach." *Journal of Family Practice* 14.3 (1982): 493–502.

Turner, Victor. *The Forest of Symbols: Aspects of Ndembu Ritual*. Ithaca, N.Y.: Cornell University Press, 1967.

———. *The Ritual Process: Structure and Anti-Structure*. Ithaca, N.Y.: Cornell University Press, 1969.

———. *Dramas, Fields, and Metaphors: Symbolic Action in Human Society*. Ithaca, N.Y.: Cornell University Press, 1974.

8. Herbal Medicine Among the Lumbee Indians

Edward M. Croom, Jr.

Among modern medical ethnobotanists there is a useful and growing tendency not to be satisfied with the mere compiling of a list of botanically identified native plant names and their uses. They seek further to assess the evidence pharmacologically and medically, or at least to present it with sufficient care to make it open to experimental verification by the appropriate scientists, whether botanists, chemists, pharmacologists, doctors, or psychiatrists.—Weston LaBarre

Introduction

The intent of this study was to document the plant remedies of the Lumbee Indians, the largest group of Indians east of the Mississippi River.[1] Few plant remedies had ever been reported for the Lumbee, and no study had ever been conducted on Lumbee herbal medicine. Indeed, no trained botanist or ethnographer has collected the plants used for medicine by any culture in eastern North Carolina during this or the previous century. Because of this lack of research, a number of remedies are documented for the first time by actual plant specimens, and a number of other medicinal uses are reported here for the first time. The primary objective was to describe as exactly and completely as possible the type of plant used for particular remedies along with the harvesting, preparation, and administration practices for the plant remedies.

Disorders most frequently mentioned as being treated by plants were fever, colds, influenza, pneumonia, measles, sores, and swellings. Plants used by the most consultants were Pine (*Pinus* spp.), Rabbit Tobacco (*Gnaphalium obtusifolium*), Sassafras (*Sassafras albidum*), Oak (*Quercus* spp.), Poke (*Phytolacca americana*), Wild Horehound (*Eupatorium rotundifolium*),

John-the-Worker (*Hypericum hypericoides*), and Salty Berry (*Rhus* spp.). Families with a large number of genera used were Asteraceae (Aster), Euphorbiaceae (Poinsettia), Lamiaceae (Mint), and Liliaceae (Lily). Many of the species contain active compounds including volatile oils, alkaloids, and tannins. Although evaluations of the safety and efficacy of the remedies are not made, pharmaceutical and toxicological data are reported from the literature. The remedies used by the Lumbee are compared for similar uses with other cultures in the southeastern United States and for the world in general. A number of the medicinal uses are considered to be unique to the Lumbee.

Ethnobotanical Research

Ethnobotany, the study of the uses of plants by people, has included investigations emphasizing cultural and symbolic aspects (Messer; Moerman 1979), folk taxonomy (Berlin et al.), ecology (Bye), and medicinal plants (Bolyard; Morton 1974; Rao).

Early notes by naturalists in the New World gave brief descriptions of useful plants. The purpose of their reports was generally to entice new settlers to America or to find new economic plants to aid the homeland's economy (Ford). Probably the most important of the early works by naturalists in the Carolinas were the reports by Lawson and Brickell. During the Civil War, Porcher published *Resources of Southern Fields and Forests*, the Confederate States' guide to useful plants, including many indigenous medicines. Not until the late nineteenth century did ethnographers begin to study systematically the medicinal plants of the American Indians. In North Carolina this involved work by Mooney ("The Sacred Formulas of Cherokees"; "Myths of the Cherokees," 1888; "Cherokee Plant Lore"; "Cherokee Theory and Practice of Medicine"; and "Myths of the Cherokee," 1898) and Mooney and Olbrechts on the Cherokee. In South Carolina work on the Catawba was done by Swanton ("Catawba Notes") and Speck ("Catawba Texts"; "Catawba Medicines"; "Catawba Herbals"). In Virginia the main tribes studied were part of the Powhatan Confederacy (Speck, *Virginia Folklore;* Speck, Hassrick, and Carpenter). More recent work on the Cherokee has been done by Banks and by Hamel and Chiltoskey. From the folklorists came Hand's monumental work, *Popular Beliefs and Superstitions from North Carolina,* which included the common names and uses of many of the state's plant remedies. Morton's work, *Folk Remedies of the Low Country,* is the only large study in the Southeast on plant remedies used by blacks.

Based mostly on inclusion in Wood et al., *Dispensatory of the United States* (USD), Mooney (1888) and Taylor evaluated the efficacy of Cherokee and Southeastern Indian remedies, respectively. Using this standard, Mooney decided that most of the remedies were ineffective. Taylor estimated that 41 percent of the remedies did not cure or alleviate the symptoms of the disease treated. Using inclusion of plants in any edition of the *United States Pharmacopoeia* or *National Formulary,* Vogel reached the conclusion that American Indians deserved a great amount of respect for their medical knowledge and had made a major contribution to scientific medicine. Although they refrained from making pharmaceutical judgments, Morton (1971) and Bolyard include comparative uses by other groups along with chemical, pharmaceutical, and toxicological information. In their study, Camazine and Bye did make medical evaluations on the Zuni Indian remedies. Recently, Daniel Moerman published a two-volume research report, *Medicinal Plants of the Native Americans,* which is a comprehensive, taxonomically validated overview of the medicinal plants reported to have been used by Native Americans. The listing of plants, compiled from various scientific and ethnographic sources, is categorized four ways: by taxon (genus and species), by indication (basic medical usage), by plant family, and by group or tribe (1:xiv). This excellent resource makes possible a more extensive comparison of Lumbee medicinal plants with those used by other Native Americans. However, Moerman does not attempt to evaluate the medical effectiveness of the plants listed. In this study, as explained later, the safety and efficacy of plants has not been determined, although pharmaceutical and toxicological data on them are reported from the literature.

The Lumbee Indians

The Lumbee are the largest group of Indians residing east of the Mississippi River. The bulk of the population today is located in Robeson County, North Carolina. The 1980 census listed 35,511 Indians in the county (U.S. Department of Commerce). The 1970 census showed that 94 percent of the Robeson County Lumbee live in rural areas and have a per capita annual income of $1,134, with 44 percent of all the Lumbee's income falling below the poverty level (Red Corn). The 1970 census also reported that in Robeson County only 17 percent of the Lumbee that are twenty-five years and older are high school graduates, with the eighth grade being the median school year completed.

The current and past struggles for Indian identity by the Lumbee are documented in books by Barton, Blu, and Dial and Eliades. Although the Lumbee have long claimed to be Indian, they have not been able to achieve recognition as an official tribe by the U.S. government. Sturtevant and Stanley (1968) suggest the problem of recognition stems from the inability to link the Lumbee to a clear antecedent tribe of Indians and the lack of Indian language and religion in the population today. Oral tradition and folklore trace Lumbee descent from the European survivors of the lost colony on Roanoke Island. Other sources suggest that the Lumbee were descendants of several Indian groups including the eastern band of Sioux, the Cherokee, and the Tuscarora. Whatever their origins, the ancestors of the present-day Lumbee made their way into the desolate swamplands surrounding the Lumber River in eastern North Carolina. There they continued to live in virtual isolation making a living by farming.

Today the Lumbee retain an Indian identity in the absence of a distinct language and religion. The Lumbee have adopted the white lifestyle and language so thoroughly that there are few remnants of Indian culture alive in their communities. Nonetheless, as Dial and Eliades write: "They are a proud people who have established their own central community of Pembroke, North Carolina, who own land and excel as farmers, established their own churches, schools and businesses. They have never been placed on reservations, nor have they been wards of either state or federal government" (xiv).

If the Lumbee do comprise a distinct ethnic group it is because of the survival of a unique body of folklore and traditions. One major body of lore linking the Lumbee to other Native Americans in the region is that concerning the use of herbal remedies to treat illness. Like many Indian groups in the United States, the Lumbee have a medical system that combines the use of herbal remedies with the magical treatment of disease by conjurers. Traditional Lumbee conjurers worked spells to cure the sick, predict the future, and influence the course of interpersonal events. While most Lumbee today consult physicians and utilize scientific medicine on a regular basis, many still rely on the use of herbal remedies to both prevent disease and treat routine conditions.

The Natural Environment

The Lumbee territory in Robeson County is located on the coastal plain of North Carolina. The coastal plain includes a diversity of habitats from the dry, turkey oak-wire grass community typical of the sandhills to dense growths of grasses, herbs, shrubs, and trees of swamp forest, pocosins, and savannahs. Robeson County, where most of the Lumbee consultants live, has a flat topography with less than 50 percent of the county in forest (Clay et al.). Lumberton, the county seat, is 132 feet above sea level and located at 34° 37′ North latitude and 79° 1′ West longitude (Britt). The soils are alluvial sedimentary sands and clays overlying crystalline rocks. Britt classified the plant communities of Robeson County as: sandhills forest, pine-oak forest, savannah, pocosin, bay forest, swamp forest, and waste places. B. W. Wells's classic *The Natural Gardens of North Carolina* gives descriptions and species lists for these and other major North Carolina plant communities.

Most of the Lumbee live in rural areas with access to a number of plant communities. Most Lumbee prefer to collect plants when needed and not to store them for later use. Thus, quick and easy access to a plant is an important attribute for its use as a folk medicine by a large number of families. Probably the most accessible plants are those of disturbed areas around the home and surrounding fields, roadsides, ditches, and the edge of forests (especially swamp, bay, and pine-oak). Because of the distance from home, the less common habitats, such as pocosin or sandhills forest, are visited generally by automobile rather than on foot. Due to drainage practices in this century, former extensive areas of swampland have been turned into many acres of cultivated fields. Because of this, the amount and variety of plants available for the immediate collection as medicine have changed dramatically during the lifetime of older Lumbee.

Research Methods

Field research was conducted in Robeson County over a two-year period in 1977–78. While conducting the research, I lived with the Lumbee and so had an opportunity to observe firsthand the preparation and use of herbal remedies. I worked specifically with twenty-five Lumbee informants (twelve men and thirteen women) over the age of sixty. I interviewed them about plant use in their homes and made collecting trips with them to harvest herbs from surrounding fields and forests. When possible, the information that was recorded for each plant remedy included: plant common name; uses; when gathered; the plant part(s) used; whether the plant was used fresh or dried; preparation of the medicine—the type and amount of plant(s), solvent(s), and heat; the route of administration; the dosage form; dose—including the amount and timing; side effects; and the name of the consultant(s). In addition, information was obtained on who had used the plant and how effective the consultant judged the remedy to be.

Most of the Lumbee consultants learned plant remedies from their families and friends as a normal part of childhood. Occasionally this information was supplemented by obtaining remedies from a herb or "doctor" book. The exception to this informal learning was a practicing herbalist who had been taught remedies by his grandmother and as a youth worked part-time for Dr. H. S. Hair, an old "Indian Doctor." Dr. Hair, a white man, lived north of Cheraw, South Carolina, and specialized in treating pellagra.

The plants collected with Lumbee consultants are on deposit as voucher specimens at the North Carolina State University Herbarium (NCSC). For vascular plants, the nomenclature in Radford et al. and Bailey Hortorium Staff was followed.

The comparative section is drawn from a number of primary references for the southeastern United States and mostly secondary sources for the remainder of the United States and the world. Most of the references for the chemical, biological, pharmaceutical, and toxicological information are review papers and other secondary sources.

Lumbee Medicine

Diseases and Treatment

A large diversity of ailments affecting many of the body's organs have been treated by Lumbee plant remedies. These disorders have been arranged (table 8.1) into general scientific categories which follow, when possible, the World Health Organization's classification of diseases (World Health Organization). The plants used for each disorder are listed in Appendix A. The most widely known and utilized plant remedies are for reducing a fever, treating sores and swellings, and treating the common infectious diseases of children and adults—colds, influenza, pneumonia, and measles.

The resource pool for information on plant remedies can be divided into several distinctive levels of priority within the community. The first option when ill is to use the remedies known by the individual and his or her immediate family. A second source of information is friends and neighbors. These family and community connections make up a large

Table 8.1 Disorders Treated by Lumbee Plant Medicines

Cancer	Scabies	Venereal disease
External	Whooping cough	Respiratory System
Circulatory System	Injury/Poisons/	Allergies
Blood clots	Toxins	Asthma
Dropsy	Antidotes	Colds
Heart	Burns	Cough
Hypertension	Emetics	Influenza
Digestive System	Skin irritation/	Pneumonia
Mouth	abrasions	Skin
Pyorrhea	Snake bites	Boils/sores
Sores	Spider bites	Dandruff
Teeth cleaning	Tick bites	General and
Teething	Wounds	miscellaneous
Thrush	Muscle, Skeletal, and	skin disorders
Stomach/Intestine	Joint Disorders	Itching
Colic	Arthritis/rheumatism	Jaundice
Diarrhea	Backache	Pimples
Indigestion	Spasms	Poison ivy/poison
Laxative	Sprains	oak
Parasites	Swellings	Rash
Ulcer	Nervous System	Sunburn
Endocrine, Metabolic,	Analgesic	Symptoms
and Nutritional	Neuritis	Fever
Disorders	Sedative	Headache
Diabetes	Pharmaceutical Aid	Pain
Gout	Flavoring	Urinary System
Pellagra	Reproductive System	Bladder
General Medicine	Aphrodisiac/sex	Enuresis
Blood purifier	tonic	Kidney
Tonic	Birth control	Kidney stones
Infectious and Parasitic	Female sexual organ	Urine, retention
Diseases	and menstrual	Veterinary
Chicken pox	disorders	Intestinal parasites
General infections	Male sexual organ	Laxative
Malaria	disorders	Snake bite
Measles	Pregnancy/childbirth	Tonic

information network and are potentially a large reference group with knowledge of alternate remedies for many disorders. A third source of information, although infrequently used, is that of herbal books. The last option is to go to a specialist with a large personal knowledge of many herbal remedies. In the past, midwives, such as Aunt Cat Lowry, furnished herbal remedies for many people in the community. Today, the only Lumbee herbal specialist combines healing by prayer with a large number of plant teas. In this system each individual may only know a few remedies for diseases encountered in his or her family, but the community's collective knowledge is quite extensive.

According to many consultants, the use of plant remedies was much more extensive in the past. Today most Lumbee go to physicians and use ethical and patent medicines for treatment of diseases. The extent of the present use of herbal remedies is difficult to estimate but does occur on a regular basis. I was told of many recent cases of people using these domestic remedies for chronic conditions such as diabetes and for common infectious diseases. Many folk remedies are used only as a last resort after the patient has lost faith in the physician's treatment of the disorder.

Some of the remedies reported were the plant remedy of choice in the past but would not be used today. An example is the use of Queen's Delight (*Stillingia sylvatica*) for syphilis, a disease that all Lumbee would now have treated by a physician. A more complicated situation arises with chronic disorders like adult-onset diabetes that a physician's treatments cannot cure in a quick, dramatic fashion. Several cases of people with adult-onset diabetes were reported to me that involved the patient having a physician diagnose the disease, an herbalist recommend a plant remedy, and the patient returning to the unsuspecting physician for confirmation of the treatment's efficacy.

The prevalent belief about the causes of disease seems similar to the larger American culture, attributing them to natural causes (for example, microorganisms and injuries). The Christian belief in sin and punishment is seen by Lumbees—as by many white and black Christians—to be a factor in determining why one person and not another gets sick. Also, the Lumbee, many Christians, and the traditional Cherokee (Mooney 1898) share a belief in the existence of an herb cure for every disease, if people are able to discover them.

This study did not thoroughly question each consultant on the diagnosis or taxonomy of disease. This can present a problem in the evaluation of remedies from the scientific point of view. The Lumbee herbalist considered neuritis to be a disease that works on the muscle and, after a few years, goes to the bone and becomes arthritis. Pellagra was said to be a skin disease that was treated by some doctors as eczema. This same consultant described three types of diabetes: (1) diabetes of the blood; (2) diabetes of the kidneys—a disorder that causes an increased volume of urine; and (3) diabetes of the bone—the most severe form, sometimes necessitating amputation of a person's legs. To cure the first two types of diabetes is believed to be no harder than to cure a severe cold.

The concept of a blood purifier is still known by many older Lumbee. It is a therapeutic class used to rid the blood of impurities, many of which cause skin disorders such as boils and rashes (see chapter five for similar beliefs among southern blacks).

Basically, the diagnosis of disease is based on symptoms such as pain, swelling, congestion, unusual discharges (for example, blood or pus in urine), and diarrhea. Today most serious diseases are diagnosed by physicians. Again, the one exception to this procedure is the herbalist who, in addition to asking about symptoms, prays for guidance while passing hands close to the patient's body. When the herbalist feels a tingling sensation over the diseased part, a diagnosis can be made.

Summary of Plants Used

The Lumbee prefer common, easily accessible plant species for medicine. Of the eighty-seven species used, 75 percent are found as common or abundant plants in the wild, 8 percent are found solely as cultivated plants, and only 17 percent are infrequent or rare in the wild or must be imported from outside the county. Of the plants mentioned by the most consultants—Rabbit Tobacco (*Gnaphalium obtusifolium*), Pine (*Pinus* spp.), Sassafras (*Sassaffras albidum*), Oak (*Quercus* spp.), Poke (*Phytolacca americana*), Wild Horehound (*Eupatorium rotundifolium*), and John-the-Worker (*Hypericum hypericoides*)—all are readily available within a few minutes walk of almost all Lumbee homes.[2] This is particularly important since there is a preference for fresh (versus dried) plant material and for quick accessibility for rapid treatment of an illness soon after its onset.

A wide variety of plants are utilized including eighty-six species of vascular plants in seventy-three genera and forty-four families, plus one lichen. The plant families with the largest number of genera used are the Aster (Asteraceae) (Mooney and Olbrechts); Poinsettia (Euphorbiaceae), Mint (Lamiaceae), and Lily (Liliaceae) (Bolyard). Using Fernald's determination of whether a species is native or introduced, 80 percent of the plants used by the Lumbee are native.

Plant Beliefs and Identification

The Lumbee do not appear to have an elaborate belief system about plants. One consultant stated that all plants could be divided into male and female plants (that is, only male plants are used for men and female for women), but he did so only for a few. Hand reported this concept of male-female plants in North Carolina as have others for elsewhere in the South and the world (Hyatt; Sillitoe).

The Lumbee plant classification generally corresponds closely to the botanical one at the species or at least generic level. However, they recognize a plant taxon called "Milkweed" that is based on the presence of milky juice and includes both the latex-bearing genera *Lactuca* (Asteraceae) and *Euphorbia* (Euphorbiaceae).

A number of characteristics are utilized by the Lumbee for purposes of identification. These include color (for example, inner bark of *Alnus*, wood of *Xanthorhiza*), milky juice as just mentioned, plant height (for example, to distinguish *Gaylussacia dumosa* from *G. frondosa*), leaf shape and growth form (for example, to distinguish *Sarracenia purpurea* from *S. flava*), and odor of leaves or roots (for example, root of *Aristolochia serpentaria*).

Plant Collection

Harvesting plants is generally done just prior to making the medicine. As a rule, fresh, healthy looking growth is chosen. The exception is Rabbit Tobacco (*Gnaphalium obtusifolium*), the green leaves of which are considered somewhat poisonous. The brown leaves are the only ones gathered. Although fresh plants are generally preferred, some are gathered and dried for later uses. The plants to be dried are generally placed in a shady, well-ventilated area and then stored in the home or in a shed or other outbuilding. After collecting, plants are cleaned of spiders and insects. If roots or other below-ground parts are gathered, any dirt is shaken, brushed, or washed off. The use of above-ground parts includes leaves, twigs, tops, or buds. "Tops" are the growing tips, including stem and leaves of herbaceous or wood plants. "Buds" include the woody twig with buds.

Preparation and Administration of the Medicine

Medicines are made into teas, poultices, and salves. Most remedies are similar to drug specifics using a single species of plant. Others follow a botanical polypharmacy approach. An example is the "shotgun heart remedy" which is prepared by combining several plants (each with unique properties) to make the medicine. For teas, plants are gently boiled on a stove in a pan of water until the decoction is a dark color or until half the water is lost, a process that takes from one to two hours. The teas are taken internally in doses from one teaspoon to one quart or more, although most doses are a swallow to a cup of liquid. One consultant used one-half to three-fourths of the normal dose for those between ten and twenty years old. The tea is generally drunk hot, and the most important doses are considered the ones taken without food in the stomach before going to sleep at night and upon waking in the morning. When teas are not stored in the refrigerator, alcohol is added as a preservative.

Salves and ointments are prepared by boiling the plants in water until only a small amount of liquid remains. The decoction is then strained and the liquid combined with hog or cow fat or a commercial product such as Rosebud Salve or Vaseline Petroleum Jelly.

A standard decoction is made by folding back the plant from the growing tip or end of a branch in six- to eight-inch lengths. These tightly folded bundles are measured for different diameters. The largest amount is measured by placing the index finger on the tip of the thumb; to make the next smallest size measurement, the index finger is placed on the first joint from the tip of the thumb (between the distal and proximal phalanx); the smallest hand measurement is made with the index finger placed at the base of the thumb (proximal phalanx).

Comparison of Lumbee Medicinal Uses with Other Cultures

Since most plant species have a restricted geographical range, all comparisons of plant uses are made at the level of the genus which generally has a much broader geographical range spanning several continents. For example, *Acorus calamus* L. is used for stomachache by the Lumbee and *A. gramineus* Soland is used similarly by people in Asia.

The distribution of the medicinal uses can be arranged into several categories. First are those plant remedies that are found in many parts of the world. A large number of Lumbee remedies are in this group. As just mentioned, the genus *Acorus* is used as a carminative for stomachache by whites, blacks, and Indians in North America as well as in Europe and Asia. Other examples include *Allium* for hypertension, *Aloe* for burns, *Ariostolochia* for snakebites, and *Cladina* for sores. Some of the medicinal uses with a more limited distribution are those used only in North America or the southeastern states. *Alnus* is an example of a genus that grows in

Table 8.2 Unique Medicinal Plant Uses by the Lumbee

Genus	Disorder(s) Treated by the Lumbee	Closely Related Disorders Treated by Others
Alnus	Blood clots, mouth sores, poison oak/poison ivy, rashes, sunburn	Circulatory problems, oral infections, skin disorders
Ambrosia	Diabetes	None
Aristida	Cross vine poisoning	None
Asclepias	Diabetes	None
Ceanothus	Sprains, swellings	Astringent and antispasmodic
Chimaphila	Neuritis	None
Cirsium	Spider bites	Bites of poisonous insects and reptiles, skin disorder
Cnidosolus	Stomach ulcer (but Lumbee consultant not positive of use)	None
Cornus	Laxative	Normally for diarrhea
Datura	Tick bite	Poisonous insects and reptiles
Daucus	Colds, pneumonia, strength	None
Elaphantopus	Pneumonia	Pulmonary disorders
Eragrostis	Kidney stones and other kidney problems	None
Gelsemium	Jaundice	None
Helenium	Allergies (hay fever), asthma, diabetes	None
Ilex	Pneumonia	Upper respiratory
Juniperus	Whooping cough	Lung disorders and coughs
Liriodendron	Bladder, kidney, including Bright's disease, pellagra	Diuretic
Melia	Veterinary—laxative	Human—laxative
Myrica	Itching	Skin problems, anesthetic
Nepeta	Cut mucous in newborn baby's throat, wounds	Cut phlegm
Persea	Boils	Skin problems
Phytolacca	Asthma, stomach ulcer veterinary—intestinal worms in chickens	Human—intestinal worms
Prunus	Dandruff; veterinary—intestinal worms	Tonic to stimulate hair growth; human—intestinal worms
Pteridium	Burns	Skin problems

Table 8.2 *Continued*

Genus	Disorder(s) Treated by the Lumbee	Closely Related Disorders Treated by Others
Rhus	Pellegra	None
Ricinus	Veterinary—intestinal worms	None
Salvia	Morning sickness in pregnant women	Carminative
Sarracenia	Kidney stones	Kidney problems
Sida	Weak back, veterinary tonic	None but has been used for urinary problems, human tonic
Silphium	Swelling	Styptic, antispasmodic
Sisyrinchium	Colds, influenza, pneumonia	Cathartic
Smilacina	Halitosis	None
Sonchus	Teething	Calmative
Stillingia	Pellegra	Skin problems
Tancetum	Morning sickness in pregnant women	Carminative

North and South America, Europe, and Asia (Willis), but almost all the Lumbee medicinal uses are restricted to Indians and other groups in the southeastern United States. *Chimaphia* is another genus that is found in Europe, Asia, and the Americas (Willis), with a number of uses shared by Indians and others throughout North America, but only rarely elsewhere. Some Lumbee remedies are only shared by people in distant parts of the world. An example is the Lumbee use of *Sida* for pimples and sores—a remedy previously reported only from Asia. The similar use of a plant by such widely separated groups may be explained as independent discoveries of the remedy in Asia and in North America.

One of the surprising results of this study was the number of medicinal uses that are unique to the Lumbee. The list in table 8.2 includes remedies that are without any similar use (for example, *Ambrosia* for diabetes), those that are unparalleled for the specific disorder but have closely related uses by others (for example, *Alnus* for blood clots by Lumbee and circulatory problems by others), and uses recorded for animals that were previously only reported for people (for example, *Melia* for a veterinary laxative by the Lumbee and recorded as a human laxative by others). The list of unique uses must be judged with some caution because of the following four limitations: (1) the use may be considered unique because there was only one Lumbee consultant who may have been mistaken about the plant's use; (2) the references consulted for comparison summarized a group's uses into general categories (for example, kidney problems) so that specific disorders (for example, kidney stones) could not be identified; (3) the remedy may have been used by other groups in the area, but has never been reported; and (4) the literature on medicinal plants of the world is so large and diverse, much of it not available in English, that a group with a similar use could have been overlooked. Nonetheless, the list includes many new medicinal uses for plants, the most impressive being those which are apparently unique to the Lumbee.

Safety and Efficacy of Lumbee Remedies

In any treatment of folk medicine, one would want to know the relative safety and efficacy of each plant discussed. As mentioned in the ethnobotany section, ethnopharmacological reports have a long tradition of including information from scientific medicine to judge the safety and efficacy of folk medicine. Although one would generally assume some degree of efficacy of a particular remedy used for generations, the actual safety and efficacy are difficult to analyze. There are three basic approaches which give different levels of information in terms of completeness.

The first and simplest is an indication of its use by different groups or cultures. Those remedies used widely over the entire range of the plant or by groups not in known contact (and therefore appearing to be by independent discovery) are, by this criterion, the most likely to be efficacious. There are severe limitations to this form of proof. One limitation is the difficulty of lay people in diagnosing disease or judging effective therapy uniformly throughout the world. This task is especially difficult because the life cycles of many diseases are short and therefore self-limiting (for example, the common cold). Also most disorders show periods of time when symptoms disappear and recur (for example, arthritis pain). Considering that the best planned clinical drug trials do not show rare adverse effects or reveal errors in judgment (Feinstein 1967, 1977; Hill 1960, 1962; Melmon et al.), it is obvious that the observations of lay people are also subject to error.

The second level of analysis is a search of the chemical, pharmaceutical, and toxicological literature on plants. This scientific literature yields important insights into possible, and in many cases probable, hazards and therapeutic activity. However, this level of analysis is also limited since it generally lacks two types of studies considered basic for establishing safety and efficacy for official drugs of the Western world. First are studies showing a clear dose-dependent response in more than one species of animal, and second are controlled clinical trials with human subjects. Melmon et al. gives a clear guide to the phases of drug development in the United States.

The third level of analysis is to require the same criteria as demanded of the listing of a drug in the *Dispensatory* or some official drug list. The simplest approach is to check the listing of the plant remedy in an official drug list. This approach is especially valuable when using recent official drug compendia since inclusion of a pharmaceutical agent should mean that the treatment was evaluated using stringent criteria for diagnosis of the disease, extensive laboratory testing for pharmaceutical and toxic properties, and controlled clinical trials. The problem with this approach is that the standards are too restrictive since most plant remedies have not undergone such extensive testing. In other words, omission from the current official drug lists does not necessarily mean lack of efficacy.

In this discussion of the medicinal plants of the Lumbee, judgments have not been made on most remedies because the scientific data are insufficient. The level of information needed to make a judgment on safety and efficacy varies but the dose-dependent drug response is generally considered minimal. This type of study is seen as basic because modern chemical analytical techniques are so sensitive that parts per million and billion can be detected. An herbal remedy that contains these extremely small amounts of compounds cannot be expected to be therapeutically effective. Therefore, knowing that a plant contains a compound which is therapeutically effective for the disorder should not be viewed as sufficient proof of efficacy. Judging the safety of herbal remedies requires procedures that will ensure the type and amount of chemical present in the test are the same as those of the practitioner's tea or salve. Thus, for a realistic evaluation, the plant remedies used by the Lumbee would need to be gathered, prepared, and administered as the Lumbee do to determine the combination and quantities of active ingredients and therapeutic doses.

Because of the numerous factors affecting the active compounds in the final dosage form and the increased possibility of an unknown mechanism of drug action, the testing of an herbal medicine is much more complex than comparable testing of a single, well-defined compound.

When a compound's structure is known, it is easier to predict its probable mechanism of action. With the mixture of numerous and many unidentified compounds in a crude drug or galenical, the mechanism of action is more likely to be unknown. To avoid missing new therapeutic mechanisms, Malone advocates the use of a general screen using laboratory animals for finding new prototype official drugs from natural products. This approach is appropriate for evaluating herbal medicine since it does not initially restrict—as do most pharmaceutical studies—testing to a very specific screen, which is severely limited in the types of therapeutic activity it can evaluate. The use of a number of specific screens is reserved until after the first general screen (Malone).

Poke (*Phytolacca americana*) serves as a good example of the problem of evaluating the risks and benefits of a folk remedy. Poke is a plant widely used in folk medicine and has been the subject of more scientific studies than most plants used as folk medicine. Poke has a number of poisonous properties. In humans and animals the plant has caused burning of the mouth, cramps, vomiting blood, bloody diarrhea, visual disturbances, weakened respiration, and death (Kingsbury; Lewis and Smith). Handling the plant has caused a temporary rise in leukemia-like white blood cells (Barker et al.). The known poisonous principles are triterpene saponins, protein mitogens, and oxalates (United States, *Herbal Pharmacology;* Kingsbury; Lewis and Elvin-Lewis). Even if Poke is effective for fighting infections (in general it seems lethal enough and has been reported to inhibit gram positive and negative bacteria [Cavillito]), can it be used safely? This depends on a number of factors.

The most important factors in Poke toxicity are the part used, when it is harvested, how it is prepared, and the dosage. Young leaves gathered in the spring and boiled in water have been eaten by thousands of southerners without any symptoms of acute poisoning. The changes in leukocytes may be beneficial, acting, as many practitioners believe, as a spring tonic or blood purifier to rid the blood of infections. At least theoretically, the powerful mitogenic activity of Poke also may induce permanent leukemia or other types of cancer. These great potentials of Poke as rational therapeutic agents or insidious toxins are yet to be firmly established by studies that are based on the actual details of harvest, preparation, and administration as a food or domestic remedy. This is why the first stage of evaluating herbal remedies must be by the documentation of the therapeutic details of their use. In general, only after this descriptive stage of research can the proper studies be done to answer the questions regarding safety and efficacy.

Calamus or Sweet Flag (*Acorus calamus*) is another excellent example of the complexities involved in evaluating the safety and efficacy of remedies. A number of laboratory studies and the widespread official use of *A. calamus* in Europe and Asia as a carminative show the remedy to be effective for relieving the stomach disorders treated by the Lumbee. When included as a regular part of the diet of laboratory rats, the plant's volatile oil retards growth, causes liver and heart abnormalities, and produces malignant tumors. The health concerns, especially when used for newborn infants with colic, are considerable. The remedy is effective but the safety of occasional use is unknown, and regular use, as mentioned, has proved harmful in several significant ways.

The problem of toxicity is clouded by the fact that people using herbal remedies are aware that a few remedies can cause various transient discomforts and assume there are no other untoward effects. Many acute symptoms of poisoning are easily noted by patients and practitioners. The Lumbee report griping pains from too large a dose of Purge Grass (*Sisyrinchium* spp.) and extreme skin irritation ("it sets my skin on fire") by bathing in Wicky (*Kalmia Carolina*). What is not obvious to lay practitioners is internal damage that is asymptomatic. Examples include the cancer-causing potential of sassafras tea (*Sassafras albidum*), or the kidney damage by ingesting turpentine from pines (while all the practitioner can see is increase in urine output that appears to be beneficial to their kidney problems), or the previously mentioned changes in the white blood cells caused by poke (*Phytolacca americana*).

The lack of information on adverse effects of plant remedies is due to at least two basic problems. In laboratory studies on plant drugs, the most extensive long-term trials have rarely been done to reveal problems of regular use. The human use of herbal remedies has been discouraged by the medical profession, and therefore this use of crude drugs is not reported by the patient to the disapproving physician. This in turn severely limits the normal surveillance of adverse drug effects and epidemiological studies because of the lack of medical records. Because of this void of information, the chronic toxicity of almost all herbal remedies remains unknown.

Lumbee plant remedies should be seen as the foundation of a popular medical system whose pharmaceutical agents remain largely unproven by scientific studies. The challenge for the future is to apply modern pharmaceutical analysis to such medical systems. These systems, in all probability, will be present for many generations to come.

The botanical names of all the plants used by the Lumbee are listed for every disease, disorder, and other use in Appendix A. The details concerning the uses of some of the most widely known Lumbee plant remedies are given in Appendix B.

Appendix A. Guide to Diseases, Disorders, and Uses

Abortion (see Birth Control)

Abrasions (see Skin Irritations)

Allergies–*Helenium amarum*

Analgesic–*Liatris regimontis*

Aphrodisiacs/Sex Tonics–*Eupatorium capillifolium, Lepidium virginicum*

Arthritis/Rheumatism–*Chimaphila maculata, Lycopodium flabelliforme, Pinus* spp.

Asthma–*Gnaphalium obtusifolium, Helenium amarum, Phytolacca americana*

Baby Food–*Nepeta cataria*

Backache–*Bidens frondosa, Sida rhombifolia, Tephrosia virginiana*

Birth Control (Abortion)–*Tanacetum vulgare*

Bladder–*Hypericum hypericoides, Liriodendron tulipifera, Prunus serotina, Quercus* spp., *Rhus* spp.

Blood Clots–*Alnus serrulata*

Blood Purifier–*Alnus serrulata, Asclepias rubra, Sassafras albidum*

Boils/Sores–*Alnus serrulata, Cladina subtenuis, Euphorbia maculata, Lactuca canadensis, Liriodendron tulipifera, Persea borbonia, Phytolacca americana, Polygonatum biflorum, Polypodium polypodioides, Pteridium aquilinum, Quercus* spp., *Sambucus canadensis, Sida rhombifolia, Verbascum thapsus*

Breath Freshener–*Smilacina racemosa*

Burns–*Aloe barbadensis, Pteridium aquilinum*

Cancer, External–*Datura stramonium*

Chicken Pox–*Sassafras albidum*

Childbirth (see Pregnancy/Childbirth)

Colds–*Alnus serrulata, Daucus carota, Eupatorium rotundifolium, Gnaphalium obtusifolium, Ilex opaca, Nepeta cataria, Pinus* spp., *Salvia officinalis, Sassafras albidum, Sisyrinchium* spp., *Solidago* spp., *Verbascum thapsus, Zea mays*

Colic–*Hypericum hypericoides, Nepeta cateria, Salvia officinalis*

Cough–*Gnaphalium obtusifolium*

Diabetes–*Ambrosia artemisiifolia, Asclepias rubra, Gaylussacia dumosa, Gaylussacia frondosa, Helenium amarum, Viburnum nudum*

Diarrhea–*Ilex opaca, Liquidambar styraciflua, Quercus* spp., *Salvia officinalis*

Emetic–*Ilex glabra*

Enuresis–*Rhus* spp.

Female Sexual Organs/Menstrual Disorders–*Aristolochia serpentaria, Mitchella repens, Prunus serotina, Quercus* spp., *Stillingia sylvatica, Tephrosia virginiana, Xanthorhiza simplicissima*

Fever–*Helenium amarum, Heterotheca graminifolia, Lagenaria siceraria, Liriodendron tulipfera, Pinus* spp., *Prunus serotina, Salix nigra, Sassafras albidum, Zea mays*

Flavoring–*Myrica cerifera, Solidago odora*

Gout–*Verbascum thapsus*

Headache–*Bidens frondosa*

Heart–*Acorus calamus, Alnus serrulata, Chimaphila maculata, Sassafras albidum*

Hypertension–*Allium vineale*

Indigestion/Stomach Pain–*Acorus calamus, Mentha spicata, Nepeta cataria, Phytolacca americana, Pinus* spp., *Salvia officinalis, Sarracenia purpurea, Smilacina racemosa*

Infections, General–*Chimaphila maculata, Quercus* spp.

Influenza–*Eupatorium rotundifolium, Gnaphalium obtusifolium, Ilex opaca, Pinus* spp., *Sassafras albidum, Sisyrinchium* spp., *Zea mays*

Insect Repellant–*Perilla frutescens*

Itch (See Scabies)

Itching–*Alnus serrulata, Ilex opaca, Myrica cerifera*

Intestinal Parasites (see Parasites, Intestinal)

Jaundice–*Alnus serrulata, Gelsemium sempervirens*

Kidney–*Aristolochia serpentaria, Chimaphila maculata, Hypericum hypericoides, Liriodendron tulipifera, Pinus* spp., *Prunus serotina, Quercus* spp., *Rhus* spp., *Tephrosia virginiana*

Kidney Stones–*Chimaphila maculata, Eragrostis spectabilis, Hypericum hypericoides, Sarracenia purpurea*

Laxative–*Cornus florida, Sisyrinchium* spp. (see also Veterinary Laxative)

Magical–*Eupatorium capillifolium*

Malaria–*Cornus florida*

Male Sexual Organ Disorders–*Aristolochia serpentaria, Xanthorhiza simplicissima*

Measles–*Sassafras albidum, Zea mays*

Menstrual Disorders (see Female Sexual Organs/Menstrual Disorders)

Mouth Sores–*Alnus serrulata, Xanthorhiza simplicissima*

Neuritis–*Chimaphila maculata, Gnaphalium obtusifolium, Pinus* spp.

Pain–*Liatris regimontis*

Parasites, Intestinal–*Chenopodium ambrosioides, Phytolacca americana* (see also Veterinary Parasites)

Pellagra–*Liriodendron tulipifera, Rhus* spp., *Stillingia sylvatica, Tephrosia virginiana*

Pimples–*Euphorbia maculata, Lactuca canadensis, Sida rhombifolia*

Pneumonia–*Daucus carota, Elephantopus* spp., *Gnaphalium obtusifolium, Ilex opaca, Pinus* spp., *Sisyrinchium* spp.

Poisoning, Antidote–*Aristida stricta*

Poison Ivy/Poison Oak–*Alnus serrulata, Euphorbia maculata, Lactuca canadensis*

Pregnancy/Childbirth–*Nepeta cataria, Prunus serotina, Rhus* spp., *Salvia officinalis, Tanacetum vulgare*

Pyorrhea–*Alnus serrulata, Liquidambar styraciflua, Smilacina racemosa*

Rash–*Alnus serrulata*

Rheumatism (see Arthritis/Rheumatism)

Scabies–*Kalmia carolina*

Sedative (Infant)–*Nepeta cataria*

Sexual Organs (see Female Sexual Organ Disorders and Male Sexual Organ Disorders)

Skin, General–*Chimaphila maculata, Euphorbia maculata, Hypericum hypericoides, Xanthorhiza simplicissima*

Snake Bites–*Aristolochia serpentaria* (see also Veterinary Snake Bites)

Sores (see Boils/Sores)

Spasms–*Phytolacca americana*

Spider Bites–*Cirsium repandum*

Sprains–*Ceanothus americanus, Quercus* spp., *Verbascum thapsus*

Stomachache (see Indigestion/Stomach Pain)

Stomach Ulcer–*Acorus calamus, Cnidoscolus stimulosus, Myrica cerifera, Phytolacca americana, Xanthorhiza simplicissima*

Sunburn–*Alnus serrulata*

Swellings–*Ceanothus americanus, Quercus* spp., *Sambucus canadensis, Silphium compositum, Verbascum thapsus*

Teeth Cleaning–*Nyssa sylvatica*

Teething–*Sonchus asper*

Thrush–*Alnus serrulata*

Tick Bites–*Datura stramonium*

Tonic–*Ceanothus americanus, Daucus carota, Hypericum hypericoides, Phytolacca americana, Sassafras albidum, Tanacetum vulgare, Xanthorhiza simplicissima* (see also Veterinary Tonic)

Urine/Retention–*Rhus* spp.

Venereal Disease–*Rhus* spp., *Stillingia sylvatica, Tephrosia virginiana*

Veterinary

Laxative–*Melia azedarach*

Parasites, Intestinal–*Melia azedarach, Phytolacca americana, Prunus serotina, Ricinus communis*

Snake Bites–*Euphorbia corollata, Euphorbia curtisii, Xanthium strumarium*

Tonic–*Chimaphila maculata, Sida rhombifolia*

Whooping Cough–*Juniperus virginiana*

Wounds–*Nepeta cataria, Verbascum thapsus*

Appendix B. Frequently Used Medicinal Plant Remedies of the Lumbee

Arrangement of the Material

Medicinal Plants: The plants are arranged alphabetically by species. Under each species the format is:

Lumbee Common Name(s) (frequently cited common name(s) in botanical manuals)

Latin Binomial with Authority (synonyms used in the pharmacological or older ethnobotanical literature)

Plant Family

Description: Perennial/annual; habit; deciduous/evergreen; root stock; stem; leaf arrangement; leaf type; inflorescence; flower; fruit/seed; flowering season; habitat; abundance in Robeson County; distribution in the eastern United States; status (native/introduced) in the flora.

Uses

Diseases and Disorders Treated

Preparation: This section includes information on collection, extraction, processing, storage, dosage, and route of administration of the medicinal plant.

Comparative: General disease category. *Specific disease*—The order of comparison with other groups is North America (north of Mexico): Indians, blacks, whites; South America (Mexico southward); Europe; Asia; Africa. Names and titles in parentheses refer to References at the end of this essay. The comparison is for the same plant genus used for the same disorder as the Lumbee. For example, *Acorus calamus* is used for stomachache by the

Lumbee, while the Asian species *A. graminus* is used for stomachache in China. After this summary of similar medicinal uses of the genus, there is a discussion of the pharmaceutical and poisonous properties of the species or genus.

Rabbit Tobacco (Life Everlasting, Catfoot)
Gnaphalium obtusifolium L.
Asteraceae

Description: Annual herbs 1–3 feet tall; erect stems with brown, shriveled leaves persisting into the winter, stems covered with felt-like hairs in the summer; leaves 1–3 inches long, alternate; flowers minute in whitish heads; late summer to fall; fields, pastures, disturbed areas; common; eastern U.S.; native.

Uses: Colds, flu, neuritis, asthma, coughs, pneumonia.

Preparation: Although sometimes used alone, Rabbit Tobacco is more typically combined with other plants. The plant is generally boiled for two hours or until the water is a dark coffee color. The stems and leaves are gathered after the frost in the fall or during the winter. They can be used fresh or dried at this time. Only the lower brown leaves are gathered in the spring and summer. The green leaves are considered to make a person sick unless he or she has a strong stomach.

For colds, the plant is boiled with Pine tops (*Pinus* spp.), Mullein (*Verbascum thapsus*), and Corn (*Zea mays*) fodder. Two other combinations for colds are: (1) Rabbit Tobacco, Pine, Wild Horehound (*Eupatorium rotundifolium*), and Goldenrod (*Solidago* spp.); and (2) Rabbit Tobacco, Tag Alder (*Alnus serrulata*), and Purge Grass (*Sisyrinchium* spp.). A bundle approximately 1½ inches in diameter and 6 inches long is boiled in a quart of water. The dose is ½–1 cup. The leaves of Rabbit Tobacco are chewed for coughs and colds by adults and older children. A decoction for colds, flu, or pneumonia is made with Holly (*Ilex opaca*) leaves and Pine tops added to the Rabbit Tobacco. A decoction made only of Rabbit Tobacco is drunk for neuritis. For those with asthma, a pillow stuffed with the leaves is slept on at night to prevent asthmatic attacks. The leaves should be replaced once a year.

This is one of the most popular plants used by the Lumbee. The decoction is drunk hot, as with most medicinal teas, and is said to cause profuse sweating.

Comparative: Nervous. *Neuritis*—Europe (Rubine et al.). Respiratory. *Asthma*—North America: Eastern Cherokee (Hamel and Chiltoskey) and Virginia Rappahannock Indians (Grime), South Carolina blacks (Morton 1974), North Carolina (Hand; Clark), and other whites (Bolyard; Levenson and Levenson); Asia (Botany Institute of Southern China). *Common Cold*—North America: Eastern Cherokee (Banks; Hamel and Chiltoskey), South Carolina Catawba (Speck 1937), and other southeastern Indians (Swanton 1928; Speck 1941), South Carolina blacks (Morton 1974), North Carolina whites (Clark); Asia (Botany Institute of Southern China). *Cough*—North America: Eastern Cherokee (Hamel and Chiltoskey) and other Indians (Moerman 1977; Black; Speck 1915), North Carolina blacks (Jacobs); Asia (United States, *Barefoot Doctors Manual;* Botany Institute of China). *Influenza*—North America: southeastern Indians (Speck 1941), South Carolina blacks (Morton 1974), whites (Porcher); Asia (United States, *Barefoot Doctor's Manual;* Botany Institute of China).

Gnaphalium was an unofficial remedy widely used for chest and bowel complaints in Europe and North America in the nineteenth century (Wood and Bache). The 1976 *British Herbal Pharmacopoeia* lists *G. uliginosum* L. as containing a volatile oil and being used for laryngitis, tonsillitis, quinsy, and upper respiratory congestion (*British Herbal Pharmacopoeia*). The plant drug is said to possess anticatarrhal, antiseptic, and antitussive properties. This is in contrast to the American opinion that the plant possesses little medicinal virtue (Wood et al.). No studies were cited in support of the plant's reputed properties. The plant is extremely aromatic and, as with many essential oils, may act as a mild expectorant when excreted through the lungs (Blacow).

The plant has been reported to contain toxic concentrations of nitrates (Kingsbury).

Poke (Pokeberry, Inkberry, Pigeonberry)
Phytolacca americana L. (*P. decandra* L.)
Phytolaccaceae

Description: Robust, perennial herbs to 9 feet tall; large white root; stems green, red, or purple; leaves to 1 foot long, alternate; flowers white in a drooping raceme; fruit a dark purple to black berry, round, soft, and juicy; waste areas, roadsides, disturbed habitats, fields, pastures; common; eastern U.S.; native.

Uses: Asthma, spring tonic, boils (risings), sores, intestinal worms in people or chickens, cramps, stomach ulcers.

Preparation: The young leaves are gathered in the spring and cooked for a short time in water. This "mess of greens" is eaten as a spring tonic to prevent boils (risings), and other "diseases of the blood." A sore is treated by a fresh berry being squeezed on it or a fresh root being applied to it.

The root is used for cramps (muscle spasms) in men and women. To worm chickens the root is left in their water trough. For worming themselves, people eat a mature leaf about 4–6 inches long and 2–3 inches wide.

To make Poke juice, a quart jar is filled to a little below the neck with ripe berries. Water is added until it is ½–1 inch over the fruits. The lid is attached and the jar is allowed to ferment for 2–3 weeks. The "juice" (wine) is strained and stored for later use. Taken for stomach ulcers, the dose is 1 teaspoon or a swallow 3 times a day. Too large a dose is inebriating.

Comparative: Digestive. *Parasites*—South America (Morton 1981); Asia (Perry); Africa (Watt and Breyer-Brandwijk). *Stomach Ulcers*—none.

General Medicine. *Tonic*—North America: Eastern Cherokee (Banks; Hamel and Chiltoskey) and other Indians (Moerman 1979), South Carolina (Morton 1974) and other blacks (Snow), whites (Bolyard; Kloss).

Muscles. *Spasms/Cramps*–North America: whites (Bolyard).

Respiratory. *Asthma*—none.

Skin. *Boils/Sores*—North America: Eastern Cherokee (Banks; Hamel and Chiltoskey) and other Indians (Gilmore), South Carolina (Morton 1974) and other blacks (Puckett), North Carolina (Hand; Clark), and other whites (Porcher; Krochmal and Krochmal; Kloss; Millspaugh); South America (Steggerda; Morton 1981); Europe (Grieve); Asia (Perry).

Veterinary. *Internal Parasites*—none.

The use of Poke for medicine centers around its use as a tonic or blood purifier. Although tonic is used in pharmacy to mean a medicine that increases muscle tone, in folk medicine its meaning can be identical to blood purifier. These folk medical categories are used for disorders that are considered to be caused by impurities or problems of the blood. These include skin disorders, internal infections, and rheumatism.

Poke has been shown to inhibit gram positive and negative bacteria (Cavallito). The plant is listed as a parasiticide in the *British Herbal Pharmacopoeia.*

The plant's poisonous properties are reported as triterpene saponins, protein mitogens, and oxalates (Lewis and Elvin-Lewis; United States, *Herbal Pharmacology;* Kingsbury). The highest concentration of the poisonous principle is in the root stock, with less in the leaves and stems, and least in the fruit (Hardin and Arena). A cup of Poke root tea made from 1/2 teaspoon of the powdered dried root caused bloody vomiting, bloody diarrhea, low blood pressure, and a rapid heartbeat (Lewis and Smith). Leaves have been reported to contain more than 10 percent oxalate, a compound which can combine with calcium and prevent its absorption from the diet. Over extended time at moderate doses, this lack of calcium can prove fatal (Kingsbury). The symptoms of poisoning include burning of the mouth, cramps, vomiting, diarrhea, visual disturbances, salivation, perspiration, lassitude, weakened respiration and pulse, and death (Kingsbury).

The fresh plant is said to often produce inflammation of the eyelids and skin, the juice or root decoction to cause pain when applied to abraded skin, and the dust of the dried root may irritate eyes and induce sneezing (Mitchell and Rook). Handling of the plant has caused abnormal blood cells which resemble cells produced by leukemia (Barker et al.; Blacow).

Pine
Pinus echinata Miller—(Shortleaf Pine)
Pinus palustris Miller—(Longleaf Pine)
Pinus virginiana Miller—(Virginia Pine)
Pinaceae

Description: *Pinus* spp.—Resinous, evergreen trees; foliage leaves needlelike, in bundles of 2 to 5; male and female reproductive structures in separate cones on the same tree; female cone matures to large woody cone with winged seeds; pollen shed in spring.

P. echinata—Large trees, bark rough; needles to 5 inches long in bundles of 2 (sometimes 3), straight; old fields, upland woods; frequent; New York to Florida; native.

P. palustris—Large trees; bark thin; needles to 16 inches long in bundles of 3; sandy soil; frequent; Virginia to Florida; native.

P. virginiana—Small trees; bark thin; needles to 2½ inches long in bundles of 2, twisted; dry soil, old fields; frequent; New York to Florida; native.

Uses: Colds, flu, pneumonia, fever, heartburn, arthritis, neuritis, kidney problems.

Preparation: Any of the local species of Pine are used. In general, the species gathered depends more on convenience than any other criteria. However, one person expressed a preference for Longleaf Pine (*Pinus palustris*) over the other species. The "tops" include the terminal bud, needles, and last 4–6 inches of the twig. Pinetops are commonly used as a remedy for colds, flu, and pneumonia. Although Pine may be used alone for these upper respiratory infections, it is generally used in combination with other plants. These combinations include: Mullein (*Verbascum thapsus*), Rabbit Tobacco (*Gnaphalium obtusifolium*), and Corn (*Zea mays*); Goldenrod (*Solidago* spp.), Wild Horehound (*Eupatorium rotundifolium*), and Rabbit Tobacco; Holly (*Ilex opaca*), Sweet Bay (*Persea borbonia* or *Magnolia virginiana*), and Rabbit Tobacco. The fresh tops are used throughout the year in making a tea by covering the plant parts with a pint to a quart of water and boiling for 2 hours. One person adds a small amount of whiskey and honey to the tea after it is boiled. A hot cupful may be taken 2–3 times a day but is always taken before going to bed at night. If a fever is present, the patient is covered with several blankets to promote copious perspiration.

The fresh needles are chewed for heartburn. The white rosin is scraped off the tree, rolled in wheat flour, and taken as a pill for kidney problems. A woman with back pains (believed to be caused by a kidney problem) took this remedy and was cured of the pain. The brown colored rosin is used for arthritis and neuritis.

Comparative: Digestive. *Indigestion*—North America: South Carolina Catawba (Speck

1944) and other Indians (Moerman 1977; Train et al.), North Carolina whites (Hand); Europe (Rubine et al.); Asia (*Wealth of India*).

Joint. *Arthritis/Rheumatism*—North America: Eastern Cherokee (Mahoney; Hamel and Chiltoskey) and other Indians (Moerman 1977; Train et al; Sturtevant), whites (Porcher; Kloss); South America (Morton 1981); Europe (Rubine et al.; Schauenberg and Paris); Asia (Perry; *Wealth of India*).

Nervous. *Neuritis*—North America: North Carolina whites (Hand); Europe (Rubine et al.); Asia (*Wealth of India*).

Respiratory. *Colds*—Eastern Cherokee (Banks; Hamel and Chiltoskey), South Carolina Catawba (Speck 1944), and other Indians (Moerman 1977; Vogel; Train et al.; Speck 1915), South Carolina and other blacks (Snow), North Carolina (Hand; Clark) and other whites (Porcher; Lust); Europe (Rubine et al.); Asia (Perry). *Influenza*—North America: Indians (Train et al.); Europe (Rubine et al.). *Pneumonia*—North America: North Carolina whites (Hand; Clark); Europe (Rubine et al.; Schauenberg and Paris).

Symptoms. *Fever*—North America: Eastern Cherokee (Banks; Hamel and Chiltoskey) and other Indians (Moerman 1977; Train et al.), North Carolina (Hand) and other whites (Bolyard); Europe (Rubine et al.).

Urinary. *Kidney*—North America. Eastern Cherokee (Mahoney; Hamel and Chiltoskey), Virginia Rappahannock (Speck et al.), and other Indians (Moerman 1977; Train et al.; Speck et al.; Wallis), blacks (Jordan), whites (Porcher; Kloss); South America (Morton 1981); Europe (Rubine et al.; Schauenberg and Paris).

Various species of the world's pines and their extracts have been used as official medicines. *Pinus palustris* is on the official drug lists of 12 countries (Penso). The pine oils and resins are the main articles of commerce. Scotch Pine oil from *P. sylvestris* L. and Dwarf Pine oil from *P. mugo* Turra have antiviral and antibacterial properties and have been approved for use in foods (Leung). The extract from the inner bark of White Pine (*P. strobus* L.) is still used in cough syrups, including Creomulsion (Tyler et al.; Leung).

Turpentine is extracted from *P. palustris*, *P. echinata*, and other species of pine (Trease and Evans; Osol and Farrar; Tyler). The main constituents of turpentine oil (distilled from turpentine) are the termpenes a- and b-pinene and camphene (Trease and Evans; Osol and Farrar). Small doses of turpentine oil stimulate the kidney and act as a diuretic, increasing the output of urine (Osol and Farrar). As with other volatile oils, it has been used as a carminative to relieve flatulence and as an expectorant (Osol and Farrar; Blacow). Turpentine used externally is considered to be an excellent rubefacient and counterirritant for use in arthritis and neuralgia (Osol and Farrar; Blacow). A commercial preparation called Haarlem oil or Dutch oil (a mixture of 1 part sulfurated linseed oil and 3 parts oil of turpentine) is used for rheumatism (*Merck Index;* Blacow). Dwarf Pine oil is used as an analgesic ointment (Leung). Earlier, turpentine was injected to increase the body's resistance to infection by increasing the production of leukocytes (Osol and Farrar). One of the symptoms of turpentine poisoning is an increased number of leukocytes (Osol and Farrar).

Turpentine has been reported to cause a number of cases of human poisoning. While the symptoms of poisoning vary, stupor is the most common. Other symptoms include vomiting, convulsions, irritation of the urinary tract, irregular heart beat, respiratory problems, shock, and death (Osol and Farrar). A diagnostic feature of the presence of a large amount of turpentine in the body is the odor of violets in urine (Osol and Farrar; Blacow).

Pine pollen has been reported to cause hay fever and asthma (Lewis and Elvin-Lewis; Mitchell and Rook). Pine trees, sawdust, and shavings, or the Pine products turpentine and rosin, cause dermatitis (Mitchell and Rook). Pine needles fed to cattle have caused low uterine weight, underweight calves, stillbirth, and abortion (Lewis and Elvin-Lewis; Kingsbury). If people respond the same as cattle, pregnant women using Pines for medicine may injure themselves or their fetuses. Because turpentine may produce irritation of the urinary tract, albumin and blood cells in the urine, difficult and painful urination, and inflammation of the kidney, Pine should not be used for urinary problems (Osol and Farrar; Blacow).

Oak
Quercus laevis Walter—Fork-Leaved Red Oak (Turkey Oak)
Quercus phellos L.—Red Oak (Willow Oak)
Fagaceae

Description: *Quercus* spp.—Deciduous trees; leaves alternate, unlobed or variously lobed; flowers minute; fruit an acorn.

Q. laevis—Small trees; bark dark, inner reddish; leaves 4½–20 inches long, many perpendicular to the ground, especially in seedlings, generally with 3 main lobes, bristle-tipped, thick; acorns faintly striped, cup covering ⅓ of the acorn; early spring; sterile, sandy soil; frequent; Coastal Plain Virginia to Florida; native.

Q. phellos—Medium to large trees; bark gray to reddish brown; leaves 2–4½ inches long, lance-shaped, narrow, bristle tipped; acorn with shallow, saucer-shaped cup; early spring; most soil; common; New York to Florida; native.

Uses: Kidney problems including Bright's disease, bladder problems, booster for other remedies, virus, menstrual bleeding, diarrhea, sores, sprains, and swellings.

Preparation: A number of species of the White and Red Oak groups are used as remedies. White Oaks were considered to be milder than Red Oaks by one consultant. The Oaks are considered to be very potent and the amount taken is considered critical. Although the entire branch or outer bark may be used, it is more common to use only the "sap layer" or inner bark (phloem).

For kidney and bladder problems, a bundle of the inner bark ½ inch in diameter by 6 inches long is combined with Wild Cherry (*Prunus serotina*) and Poplar (*Liriodendron tulipifera*) in a quart of water and boiled until only 3 pints remain. The dose is 1 tablespoon taken 3 times a day. Oak tea can be taken for diarrhea, which is cured after only 2 doses of 1 tablespoon each. Sores are bathed in the decoction to aid in healing.

For viruses, a decoction is made from 3 pieces of the inner bark that are 3–4 inches long placed in 2 cups of water that is boiled until 1 cup remains. Only a swallow or two is taken since too large a dose is constipating. Another consultant commented that pure lye could be made from Red Oaks, implying the need for caution in using such a potentially caustic plant.

A tea from the sap layer is also taken to stop menstrual bleeding. The branches from Red or White Oaks are combined with other plants to increase the potency (as a booster) of other medicines. Swellings and sprains are treated with a poultice made of the inner bark from Oak, the leaves from Mullein (*Verbascum thapsus*), and the root from Red Shank (*Ceanothus americanus*).

Comparative: Digestive. *Diarrhea*—North America: Eastern Cherokee (Mooney and Olbrechts; Banks; Hamel and Chiltoskey), Southeastern Houma (Moerman 1977), and other Indians (Moerman 1977; Black), South Carolina (Morton 1974) and other blacks (Lust), North Carolina (Clark) and other whites (Kloss); South America (Morton 1981); Europe (Grieve; Rubine et al.; *British Herbal Pharmacopoeia*); Asia (Perry; *Wealth of India;* Leung); Africa; (Watt and Breyer-Brandwijk).

Infection. *Viral*—North America: Indians (for colds) (Gilmore), South Carolina blacks (Morton 1974), whites (Kloss).

Muscle. *Sprain*—Europe (Rubine et al.) *Swelling*—North America: Southeastern Houma Indians (Speck 1941), whites (Kloss); Europe (Rubine et al.).

Pharmaceutical Aid. *Booster*—North America: Southeastern Houma Indians (for tonic) (Speck 1941); Europe (Rubine et al.).

Reproductive. *Menstrual Problems*—North America: Eastern Cherokee Indians (Banks), South Carolina blacks (Levenson and Levenson), whites (Lust; Kloss; Brickell); Europe (Rubine et al.); Asia (Perry).

Skin. *Sores*—North America: Florida Seminole (Sturtevant), southeastern Alabama (Taylor), and other Indians (Moerman 1977; Gilmore; Swanton 1928), North Carolina (Hand; Bruton) and other whites (Bolyard; Lust; Kloss); Europe (Rubine et al.); Asia (Perry; Leung).

Urinary. *Bladder*—North America: Eastern Cherokee Indians (Mooney and Olbrechts), whites (Kloss); Europe (Rubine et al.); Asia (*Wealth of India;* Leung).

The Lumbee uses follow the past official medical belief that Oaks are antiseptic (useful for infections) and astringent (useful for reducing swellings, stopping secretions, and bleeding). The *Dispensatory* of 1839 listed Oak bark from *Q. alba* L. and other species as an official remedy for external ulcers, chronic diarrhea, infant cholera, scrofula (tuberculosis), and leukorrhea (Wood and Bache). White Oak, *Q. alba*, was in the *U.S. Pharmacopeia* from 1820–1900 (Bolyard).

The tannin quercitannic acid composes 6–11 percent of the bark of White Oak. The glycoside quercitrin is present and on hydrolysis yields quercetin. Other compounds from Oaks include tannic acid, methysalicylate, and shikimic acid (reported to be a mutagen, tumor producer, and carcinogen) (*Registry of Toxic Effects;* Trease and Evans; Osol and Farrar; *Merck Index*).

Tannins have shown antiviral and antimicrobial activity, but also have been implicated in human cancers (Leung). Tannic acid (or possibly a contaminant) has been thought to cause fatal liver damage when applied to extensive areas of burns or as an ingredient in enemas (Leung). Ingestion of large amounts of tannins has caused gastric irritation, nausea, and vomiting (Leung). Oaks probably vary considerably in their ability to cause poisoning. The use of *Q. alba* in past official medicine and its preference by one Lumbee consultant may reflect its lower toxicity than other species, especially the Red Oaks. Methyl salicylate is used in official medicine as a counterirritant but can also cause severe poisoning (*Merck Index*).

Sassafras, Sassafrax, Red Sassafras, White Sassafras
Sassafras albidum (Nutall) Nees (*Laurus sassafras* L., *S. officinale*
Nees et Eberm., *S. variifolium* (Salisb.) Kuntze
Lauraceae

Description: Deciduous, aromatic, small trees or shrubs; twigs, green, bark thick and furrowed when mature; leaves 2½–5 inches long, alternate, either unlobed, lobed on 1 side, or 3-lobed; flowers small, yellow in clusters at the end of twigs; fruit a dark blue fleshy drupe on a bright red stalk and cup; early spring; fence-rows, woodland borders, old fields; common; eastern U.S.; native.

Uses: Measles, chicken pox, colds, flu, "shotgun heart remedy," fever, blood purifier, spring tonic.

Preparation: This is one of the most popular remedies used by the Lumbee. The "red root" (root with red bark) is generally used. One person believed that the "white root" (root with white bark) would "run you blind." Another person thought the red was better than the white "when the white blood cells were trying to get in control."

The root is gathered anytime during the year it is needed. Two large handfuls are placed in 2–3 quarts of water and boiled until only 1 quart remains. At night a child with measles or chicken pox is given 1 pint of the tea to drink as hot as the child can tolerate. After going to bed the child is covered with heavy quilts and blankets to promote copious perspiration. It is claimed that by morning the measles are broken out, the child feels better, and any fever is gone. Adults or children with colds or flu are treated in the same manner as for children with measles.

For a blood purifier or spring tonic, Sassafras has been used in the belief it will prevent diarrhea, sores, pimples, and high or low blood pressure. Especially in the past, many children were given several glassfuls of tea for 3 or 4 consecutive nights every spring and fall.

Red Sassafras is also used in a "shotgun heart remedy" with White Garlet (identity unknown), Calmy (*Acorus calamus*), and Pip (*Chimaphila maculata*). Presumably Sassafras is included in the remedy to rid the blood of any impurities. (See *Acorus calamus.*)

The flavor of Sassafras is enjoyed so much that it is drunk by many people purely as a tasty beverage and by some as root beer.

Comparative: Circulatory. *Heart*—North America: southeastern Indians (Taylor).

General Medicine. *Blood Purifier*—North America: Eastern Cherokee (Mahoney; Banks; Hamel and Chiltoskey), southeastern (Taylor), and other Indians (Moerman 1977; Gilmore; Fenton), blacks (Puckett; Snow), North Carolina (Hand) and other whites (Bolyard; Lawson; Lust; Kloss; Brickell; Ashe); Europe (Grieve). *Tonic*–North America: Virginia Rappahannock (Speck et al.) and other Indians (Moerman 1977; Black; Penso; Speck 1915), South Carolina (Moerman 1974) and other blacks (Snow), whites (Bolyard; Kloss; Wilson); Europe (Grieve).

Infectious. *Chicken Pox*—North America: blacks (Jordan), whites (Hand). *Measles*—North America: Virginia Rappahannock (Speck et al.) and other southeastern Indians (Taylor; Speck 1941), South Carolina (Moerman 1974) and other blacks (Jordan), North Carolina (Hand; Clark) and other whites (Porcher), Louisiana (no race given) (Roberts).

Respiratory. *Common Cold*—North America: Eastern Cherokee (Banks; Hamel and Chiltoskey) and Florida Seminole Indians (Sturtevant), North Carolina (Clark) and other whites (Bolyard; Porcher). *Influenza*—North America: whites (Lawson).

Symptoms. *Fever*—North America: Eastern Cherokee (Mahoney), Virginia Rappahannock (Speck et al.), Florida Seminole (Sturtevant), and other Indians (Moerman 1977; Felter; Fenton; Speck 1915), whites (Porcher; Barton); Europe (Fenton).

During the early exploration of the New World, Sassafras is credited with raising more interest in Europe than tobacco or any other American crop (Vogel). Hariot, reporting in 1587 on the commodities of the North Carolina and Virginia area, said that Sassafras, called Winauk by the Indians, was a cure for many diseases (Corbitt). Gerarde mentions its use in England by the end of the sixteenth century (Flückiger and Hanbury). The root bark was listed in the *United States Pharmacopoeia* from 1820–1926 (Vogel). The uses of Sassafras revolve around its reputed therapeutic properties as a diaphoretic and alterative, blood purifier, or tonic. These attributes would recommend its use to reduce a fever and help cleanse the blood of infections.

The root bark yields from 3–9 percent oil (which is 80–90 percent safrole, approximately 7 percent *d*-camphor, and 0.5–6.5 percent eugenol), approximately 6 percent tannin, approximately 9 percent phlobaphene, resin, and starch (Osol and Farrar; *Wealth of India; British Herbal Pharmacopoeia*). Other compounds from the plant include a- and b-pinene, asarone, thujone, a sesquiterpene, phellandrene, and phenol (Bolyard; Claus et al.; *Wealth of India;* Leung). Several of these compounds act as anti-infectives and irritants to the mucous membranes as do volatile oils in general (Lewis and Elvin-Lewis; Blacow). Sassafras oil was used in official medicine as a disinfectant for root canals, to destroy head lice, for nasal congestion, and generally was considered to be a powerful antiseptic (Osol and Farrar).

The oil given to experimental animals caused death by fatty degeneration of tissues including the liver, kidneys, and heart, or by depression of circulation and respiratory paralysis (Osol and Farrar). Even a single teaspoon of the oil taken by a young man was reported to cause vomiting, dilated pupils, and stupor (Osol and Farrar). The larger problem of safe use of Sassafras revolves around its cancer-causing potential from small doses over long periods of time. Based on its safrole content, Segelman et al. have made a strong case for the potential of Sassafras tea to cause cancer. Some laboratory studies with rats show that safrole must be metabolized to 1′-hydroxysafrol to cause cancerous growths (Tyler). In rats and human subjects, small doses of safrole have not yielded 1′-hydroxysafrole in the urine and almost all the safrole was excreted within 24 hours (Bolyard; Tyler). With large doses (750 mg/kg) 1′-hydroxysafrole was found in the rat but not human urine (Tyler), raising the question of the reality of the human cancer risk in using Sassafras. However, one study has shown safrole-free extracts to produce tumors (Tyler et al.). Safrole has been banned by the FDA as a food additive because of its potential as a carcinogen (Tyler et al.).

Notes

1. This chapter is based on the knowledge of the twenty-five Lumbee Indians who freely shared their personal heritage and direct experiences with me. A special thanks for sharing many of these remedies is due to Vernon Cooper, Annie Mae Oxendine, and Willie French Thompson. Because the research was conducted as a doctoral dissertation, my graduate committee, James W. Hardin, Jon M. Stucky, Richard A. Yarnell, and Jack K. Weir, offered a great range and depth of guidance.

2. Interestingly, none of these is found on Moerman's list of the ten most used species of medicinal plants among Native Americans (1:xiv), although it does include a different pine species, *Pinus strobus.*

References

Ashe, T. "Carolina, or a Description of the Present State of that Country." *Narratives of Early Carolina, 1605–1708.* Ed. A. S. Salley, Jr. New York: Chas. Scribner's Sons, 1911. 136–69.

Bailey Hortorium Staff. *Hortus Third.* New York: MacMillan, 1976.

Banks, W. H., Jr. "Ethnobotany of the Cherokee Indians" Dissertation. University of Tennessee, 1953.

Barker, B. E., P. Farnes, and H. Fanger. "Mitogenic Activity in Phytolacca Americana." *Lancet* 1 (1965): 170.

Barton, L. R. *The Most Ironic Story in American History.* Charlotte, N.C.: Associated Printing, 1967.

Berlin, B., D. E. Breedlove, and P. H. Raven. *Principles of Tzeltal Plant Classification: An*

Introduction to the Botanical Ethnography of a Mayan-Speaking People of the Highland Chiapas. New York: Academic, 1974.

Black, M. J. *Algonquin Ethnobotany: An Interpretation of Aboriginal Adaptation in Southwestern Quebec.* Canadian Ethnology Service, National Museum of Man Mercury Series 65. Ottawa: National Museums of Canada, 1980.

Blacow, N. W., ed. *Martindale: the Extra Pharmacopoeia.* 26th ed. London: Pharmaceutical, 1972.

Blu, K. I. *The Lumbee Problem: The Making of an American Indian People.* New York: Cambridge University Press, 1980.

Bolyard, J. C. *Medicinal Plants and Home Remedies of Appalachia.* Springfield, Ill.: C. C. Thomas, 1981.

Botany Institute of Southern China. *Colored Atlas of Chinese Herb Medicine.* Guangzhou, China: Academy Sinica, 1977.

Brickell, J. *The Natural History of North Carolina.* 1737. Murfreesboro, N.C.: Johnson, 1963.

British Herbal Pharmacopoeia. London: British Herbal Medicine Association, 1976–79.

Britt, R. F. "The Vascular Flora of Robeson County, NC." Dissertation. University of North Carolina, 1960.

Bruton, H. S. "Miscellaneous Beliefs and Home Remedies." *North Carolina Folklore* 1.1 (1948): 20–26.

Bye, R. A. "Quelites: Ethnoecology of Edible Greens—Past, Present, and Future." *Journal of Ethnobiology* 1 (1981): 109–23.

Camazine, S., and R. A. Bye. "A Study of the Medical Ethnobotany of the Zuni Indians of New Mexico." *Journal of Ethnopharmacology* 2 (1980): 365–88.

Cavallito, C. J. "Antibiotics from Plants." *Medicinal Chemistry: A Series of Reviews.* Vol. 1. Ed. C. M. Suter. New York: Wiley, 1951.

Clark, J. D. "North Carolina Popular Beliefs and Superstitions." *North Carolina Folklore* 18.1 (1970): 1–67.

Claus, E. P., V. E. Tyler, and L. R. Brady. *Pharmacognosy.* 6th ed. Philadelphia: Lea, 1970.

Clay, J. W., D. M. Orr, Jr., and A. W. Stuart, eds. *North Carolina Atlas: Portrait of a Changing State.* Chapel Hill: University of North Carolina Press, 1975.

Corbitt, D. L., ed. *Descriptions and Attempted Settlements of Carolina, 1684–1590.* Revised ed. Raleigh, N.C.: State Department of Archives and History, 1953.

Dial, A. L., and D. K. Eliades. *The Only Land I Know: A History of the Lumbee Indians.* San Francisco: Indian Historian, 1975.

Feinstein, A. R. *Clinical Judgement.* Baltimore: Williams, 1967.

———. *Clinical Biostatics.* St. Louis, Mo.: Mosby, 1977.

Felter, H. W. *The Genesis of the American Materia Medica.* Bulletin 26, Series 8. Cincinnati: Lloyd Library, 1927.

Fenton, W. N. *Contacts Between Iroquois Herbalism and Colonial Medicine.* Smithsonian Annual Report no. 194. Washington, D.C.: GPO, 1941.

Fernald, M. L. *Gray's Manual of Botany.* 8th ed. New York: American, 1980.

Flückiger, A., and D. Hanbury. *Pharmacographia: A History of the Principal Drugs of Vegetable Origin Met with in Great Britain and British India.* London, 1879.

Ford, R. I. "Ethnobotany: 'Historical Diversity and Synthesis.'" *The Nature and Status of Ethnobotany.* Ed. R. I. Ford. Ann Arbor: University of Michigan Press, 1978. 33–49.

Gilmore, M. R. "Uses of Plants by the Indians of the Missouri River Region." *Bureau of American Ethnology,* 33d Annual Report. Washington, D.C.: Smithsonian, 1919. 43–164.

Grieve, M. *A Modern Herbal.* New York: Dover, 1971. Originally published in 1931 by Harcourt, Brace & Co., New York.

Grime, W. E. *Botany of the Black Americas.* St. Clair Shores, Mich.: Scholarly, 1976.

Hamel, P. B., and M. U. Chiltoskey. *Cherokee Plants and Their Uses—A 400-Year History.* Sylva, N.C.: Herald, 1975.

Hand, W. D., ed. *Popular Beliefs and Superstitions from North Carolina.* Vol. 6 of *The Frank C. Brown Collection of North Carolina Folklore.* Durham, N.C.: Duke University Press, 1961.

Hardin, J. W., and J. M. Arena. *Human Poisoning from Native and Cultivated Plants.* 2d ed. Durham, N.C.: Duke University Press, 1973.

Hill, A. B. *Statistical Methods in Clinical and Preventive Medicine.* Edinburgh: E. & S. Livingstone, Ltd., 1962.

———. *Controlled Clinical Trials.* Conference of Council for International Organization of Medical Sciences. Oxford: Blackwell, 1960.

Hyatt, H. M. *Hoodoo—Conjuration—Witchcraft—Rootwork.* Hannibal, Mo.: Western, 1970.

Jacobs, M. "Black Remedies and Cures." *Kin'lin'* (Hallsboro, N.C., 1975): 18–19.

Jordan, W. C. "Voodoo Medicine." *Textbook of Black-Related Diseases.* Ed. R. A. Williams. New York: McGraw-Hill, 1975.

Kingsbury, J. M. *Poisonous Plants of the United States and Canada.* Englewood Cliffs, N.J.: Prentice-Hall, 1964.

Kloss, J. *Back to Eden.* Santa Barbara, Calif.: Lifeline, 1974.

Krochmal, A., and C. Krochmal. *A Guide to the Medicinal Plants of the United States.* New York: Quadrangle, 1973.

LaBarre, Weston. "Materia medica of the Aymara, Lake Titicaca Plateau, Bolivia." *Webbia* 15 (1990): 47–94.

Lawson, J. *A New Voyage to Carolina.* 1709. Chapel Hill: University of North Carolina Press, 1967.

Leung, A. Y. *Encyclopedia of Common Natural Ingredients Used in Food, Drugs, and Cosmetics.* New York: Wiley, 1980.

Levenson, B., and M. H. Levenson. "Some Southern Folk Remedies and Related Beliefs." *North Carolina Folklore* 8.2 (1960): 26–31.

Lewis, W. H., and M. P. F. Elvin-Lewis. *Medical Botany.* New York: John Wiley & Sons, 1977.

Lewis, W. H., and P. R. Smith. "Poke Root Herbal Tea Poisoning." *Journal of the American Medical Association* 242 (1979): 2,759–60.

Lust, J. *The Herb Book.* New York: Bantam, 1974.

Mahoney, J. W. *The Cherokee Physician or Indian Guide to Health as Given by Richard Foreman.* 1857. 3d ed. James M. Edney, New York. Hooper reprint, Norman, Okla., 1975.

Malone, M. H. "The Pharmacological Evaluation of Natural Products—General and Specific Approaches to Screening Ethnopharmaceuticals." *Onderzoek naar Biologische Aktiviteit van Natuurstofen.* Proceedings van het 7de Symposium voor farmacognisie. Ed. C. Violon, V. Maes, and A. Vercruysse. Brussels: Vrije Universiteit Brussel, 1981.

Melmon, K. E., A. G. Gilman, and S. E. Mayer. "Principles of Therapeutics." *The Pharmacological Basis of Therapeutics.* 6th ed. Ed. A. G. Gilman, L. S. Goodman, and A. Gilman. New York: Macmillan, 1980. 40–55.

Merck Index. 9th ed. Ed. M. Windholz. Rahway, N.J.: Merck, 1976.

Messer, E. "Present and Future Prospects of Herbal Medicine in a Mexican Community." *The Nature and Status of Ethnobotany.* Ed. R. E. Ford. Ann Arbor: University of Michigan Press, 1978. 137–61.

Millspaugh, C. F. *Medicinal Plants.* 1892. Reprinted as *American Medicinal Plants.* New York: Dover, 1974.

Mitchell, J., and A. Rook. *Botanical Dermatology.* Vancouver: Greenglass, 1979.

Moerman, D. E. "Extended Family and Popular Medicine on St. Helena Island, S.C.: Adaptations to Marginality." Dissertation. University of Michigan, 1974.

———. *American Medical Ethnobotany.* New York: Garland, 1977.

———. "Symbols and Selectivity: A Statistical Analysis of Native American Ethnobotany." *Journal of Ethnopharmacology* 1 (1979): 111–19.

———. *Medicinal Plants of the Native Americans.* 2 vols. Technical Reports 16. Ann Arbor: University of Michigan Museum of Anthropology, 1986.

Mooney, J. "The Sacred Formulas of the Cherokees." *Bureau of American Ethnology.* Smithsonian. 7th Annual Report. Washington, 1886, 301–97.

———. "Myths of the Cherokees." *Journal of American Folklore* 1.2 (1888): 97–108.

———. "Cherokee Plant Lore." *American Anthropology* 2 (1889): 223–24.

———. "Cherokee Theory and Practice of Medicine." *Journal of American Folklore* 3 (1890): 44–50.

———. "Myths of the Cherokee." *Bureau of American Ethnology.* Smithsonian. 19th Annual Report. Washington, 1898.

Mooney, J., and F. M. Olbrechts. "The Swimmer Manuscript: Cherokee Sacred Formulas and Medicinal Prescriptions." *Bureau of American Ethnology.* Smithsonian. Bulletin 99. Washington, D.C.: GPO, 1932.

Morton, J. F. *Folk Remedies of the Low Country.* Miami: Seemann, 1974.

———. *Atlas of Medicinal Plants of Middle America.* Springfield, Ill.: Thomas, 1981.

Osol, A., and G. E. Farrar, eds. *The Dispensatory of the United States of America.* 25th ed. Philadelphia: Lippincott, 1955.

Penso, G. *Inventory of Medicinal Plants and Compilation of a List of the Most Widely Used Plants.* DPM 78.2. Geneva: WHO, 1978.

Perry, L. M. *Medicinal Plants of East and Southeast Asia: Attributed Properties and Uses.* Cambridge, Mass.: MIT Press, 1980.

Porcher, F. P. *Resources of the Southern Fields and Forests.* 1863. New York: Arno, 1970.

Puckett, N. N. *Folk Beliefs of the Southern Negro.* 1926. University of North Carolina Press, Chapel Hill. Negro University Press reprint, New York, 1968.

Radford, A. E., H. E. Ahles, and C. R. Bell. *Manual of the Vascular Flora of the Carolinas.* Chapel Hill: University of North Carolina Press, 1968.

Rao, R. R. "Ethnobotany of Meghalaya: Medicinal Plants Used by Khasi and Garo Tribes." *Economic Botany* 35 (1981): 4–9.

Red Corn, J. *American Indians of the South Atlantic Region by County.* Prepared for Community Services Administration by American Indian Census and Statistical Data Project. Publication no. 82-102070. Springfield, Va.: National Technological Information Service, 1980.

Registry of Toxic Effects of Chemical Substances: Cincinnati: National Institute for Occupational Safety and Health, 1977.

Roberts, H. "Louisiana Superstitions." *Journal of American Folklore* 40 (1927): 144–208.

Rubine, H., S. Ozola, and V. Enina. *Arstniecibas augu Sagatavosama un Lietosana.* (*Preparation and Use of Medicinal Plants*). Riga, Latvia: Zvaigzne, 1974.

Schauenberg, P., and F. Paris. *Guide to Medicinal Plants.* Trans. M. Pugh-Jones. New Canaan, Conn.: Keats, 1977.

Segelman, A. B., F. P. Segelman, J. Karliner, and R. D. Sofia. "Sassafras and Herb Tea: Potential Health Hazard." *Journal of the American Medical Association* 236.5 (1976): 477.

Sillitoe, P. "The Gender of Crops in the Papua, New Guinea Highlands." *Ethnology* 20 (1981): 1–14.

Snow, L. F. "The Medical System of a Group of Urban Blacks." Dissertation. University of Arizona, 1971.

———. "Catawba Herbals and Curative Practices." *Journal of American Folklore* 52 (1944): 37–50.

———. "Catawba Medicines and Curative Practices." *Publication of the Phil. Anthropological Society* 1 (1937): 179–97.

———. "Catawba Texts." *Columbia University Contributions in Anthropology* 24 (1934): 1–91.

———. "A List of Plant Curatives Obtained from the Houma Indians of Louisiana." *Primitive Man* 14.4 (1941): 49–73.

Speck, F. G. "Medicine Practices of the Eastern Algonquins." Proceedings of the 19th International Congress of Americanists. Washington, D.C.: 1915. 303–21.

———. *Virginia Folklore and Medical Practices.* Philadelphia: n. p., n. d.

Speck, F. G., R. B. Hassrick, and E. S. Carpenter. "Rappahannock Herbals, Folk-lore and Science of Cures." Proceedings of the Delaware County Institute of Science 10 (1942): 7–55.

Steggerda, M. "Some Ethnological Data Concerning One Hundred Yucatan Plants." Smithsonian. *Bureau of American Ethnology Bulletin* 136 (1943): 189–226.

Sturtevant, W. C. "The Mikasuki Seminole: Medical Beliefs and Practices." Dissertation. Yale University, 1955.

Sturtevant, W. C., and S. Stanley. "Indian Communities in the Eastern States." *Indian Historian* 1 (1968): 15–19.

Swanton, J. R. "Catawba Notes." *Journal of the Washington Academy of Science* 8 (1918): 623–29.

———. "Religious Beliefs and Medical Practices of the Creek Indians." *Bureau of American Ethnology.* Smithsonian. 42d Annual Report. Washington, D.C.: GPO, 1928. 472–672.

Taylor, L. A. *Plants Used as Curatives by Certain Southeastern Tribes.* Cambridge, Mass.: Botanical Museum of Harvard University, 1940.

Train, P., J. R. Henrichs, and W. A. Archer. *Medicinal Uses of Plants by Indian Tribes of Nevada.* Division of Plants Exploration and Introduction, Bureau of Plant Industry, USDA. Publication # 33. Washington, D.C.: GPO, 1941.

Trease, G. E., and W. C. Evans. *Pharmacognosy.* 11th ed. London: Bailliere, 1978.

Tyler, V. E. *The Honest Herbal.* Philadelphia: Stickley, 1982.

Tyler, V. E., L. R. Brady, and J. E. Robbers. *Pharmacognosy.* 8th ed. Philadelphia: Lea and Febiger, 1981.

United States, Department of Commerce, Bureau of the Census. *North Carolina Final Population and Housing Unit Counts.* PHC 80-V-35. Washington, D.C.: GPO, 1982.

United States, J. E. Fogarty International Center for Advanced Study in Health Science. *A Barefoot Doctor's Manual.* Washington, D.C.: GPO, 1974.

United States, National Academy of Sciences. *Herbal Pharmacology in the People's Republic of China—a Trip Report of the American Herbal Pharmacology Delegation.* Washington, D.C.: GPO, 1975.

Vogel, V. J. *American Indian Medicine.* Norman: University of Oklahoma Press, 1970.

Wallis, W. O. "Medicines Used by the Micmac Indians." *American Anthropologist* 24 (1922): 24–30.

Watt, J. M., and M. G. Breyer-Brandwijk. *Medicinal and Poisonous Plants of Southern and Eastern Africa.* 2d ed. Edinburgh: E. & S. Livingstone Ltd., 1962.

Wealth of India. Raw Materials Series 1948–76. New Delhi: Council of Scientific and Industrial Research, n.d.

Wells, B. W. *The Natural Gardens of North Carolina.* Chapel Hill: University of North Carolina Press, 1967.

Willis, J. C. *A Dictionary of the Flowering Plants and Ferns.* 8th ed. revised. Cambridge: Cambridge University Press, 1973.

Wilson, G. "Local Plants and Folk Remedies in the Mammoth Cave Region." *Southern Folklore Quarterly* 32 (1968): 320–27.

Wood, G. B., and F. Bache. *The Dispensatory of the United States of America.* 4th ed. Philadelphia: Grigg and Elliot, 1839.

Wood, H. C., Jr., C. H. LaWall, H. W. Youngken, A. Osol, I. Griffith, and L. Gershenfeld, eds. *The Dispensatory of the United States of America.* 22d ed. Philadelphia: Lippincott, 1937.

World Health Organization. *Manual of the International Statistical Classification of Diseases, Injuries, and Causes of Death 1977–1978.* 9th ed. revised. Geneva: WHO, n.d.

9. Childbirth Education and Traditional Beliefs About Pregnancy and Childbirth

C. W. Sullivan III

In spite of the scientific and medical advances of the last few centuries (up to and including the recent "test-tube" babies), the events of conception, pregnancy, and childbirth have remained mysterious and/or wonderful to most people. A part of the mystery, certainly, arises from the general public's lack of information about what actually goes on, especially during pregnancy and childbirth. As a result, the woman and the fetus have often received less than the best possible care in these situations. Women have, of course, been bombarded with a great deal of advice—sound and otherwise—concerning their own care and the care of the unborn child. Fortunately, however, professional medicine and women's rights groups have recently combined to present childbirth education classes which dispel some of the mystery, much of the ignorance, and hopefully, most of the fear.

There has always been a good deal of folklore surrounding pregnancy and childbirth. Baby showers, the selection of possible names, the pink or blue color scheme, and the passing out of cigars are among the customary traditional activities which attend a child's birth. Folk speech and naming not only govern the selection of a child's name, but also allow people to talk about "bundles of joy," "arrivals from heaven," and the coming of "the stork." And handcrafted quilts, cradles, and christening gowns are among the items passed from generation to generation. From a medical standpoint, however, the most interesting traditions may involve the folk beliefs which surround pregnancy and childbirth. Such folk beliefs exist among those women who have taken childbirth education courses as well as among those who have had no such instruction. The purpose of this study is to survey and comment on the folk beliefs recounted by women who have taken part in childbirth education courses.

Historically, the cultural and social position of the pregnant woman in Western Europe and European North America has varied considerably from age to age, and it is interesting that the mysterious ability to bear young, the characteristic which made the female the first deity (the Earth Mother) over 30,000 years ago, fell subsequently upon such hard times. Although female midwives (who had done that job for centuries) were still as knowledgeable and capable as anyone in the delivering of babies, they began to be displaced by male midwives and obstetricians who began to take over as supervisors of the birth process in the early years of the seventeenth century (Donegan 19). This, however, was only the final stage of a process begun centuries earlier. In fact, the establishment of maternity hospitals in fourteenth-century Europe may be the historical point from which the rise of the male midwife and, later, the obstetrician can be charted (Thoms 14). The growing acceptance of men in the lying-in room (as religious objections were relaxed), the spread of medical schools and hospitals, the development of anesthesia, and other medical and cultural changes allowed men to equal women in the delivery rooms of Europe and almost completely displace the midwife for women in the middle and upper classes in the United States by the early years of the twentieth century (Thoms 17).

The movement of men into this previously female-dominated area was by no means smooth and steady. Some very interesting things happened along the way, including fierce propaganda wars waged by both sides. In 1522 in Germany, "a Dr. Wertt was burned at the stake for attending childbirth disguised as a woman." Francis Rayus, arrested for the same crime in Wells, Massachusetts, in 1646, was only fined fifty shillings (Donegan 18). Even stranger, perhaps, is the story of the Chamberlen family which, in the sixteenth and seventeenth centuries, invented the forceps and then kept them a family secret for several generations (Cutter and Viets 44–55). The propagandistic (and not necessarily factual) accounts of errors—by midwives and doctors alike—are quite gruesome. Nineteenth-century medical journals related stories of midwives who "might have torn out the patient's womb, pulled the child's body from its head, or perpetrated lesser, but nevertheless permanent, injuries on both mother and child." And the same journals also told of "male practitioners who in their ignorance had actually cut out the womb, or part of the intestines, with scissors or knife" (Donnison 56).

It is no wonder that against such a background certain traditional folk characters appeared. One such, the drinking female midwife, is referred to by Toby Belch in Shakespeare's *Twelfth Night* (II.v.216) and is such a prominent stereotype that eighteenth- and nineteenth-century advocates of midwifery felt compelled to refute the image in no uncertain terms (Donnison 33–34). And the clumsy and unsympathetic doctor, with his cold and insensitive metal instruments, may not yet have had his image redeemed. The male midwife is certainly a humorous character in Sterne's *Tristram Shandy*. Dr. Slop, a caricature of the well-known Dr. Burton of York, first belittles the midwife who has called him in to help with the delivery and then, mishandling his forceps, crushes the bridge of baby Tristram's nose (Donnison 29). The modern belief that only those male students who cannot make it in any other field of medicine become obstetricians and gynecologists may well be descended from the figures on whom Dr. Slop was based.

When the male doctors finally took over from the midwives in the United States, it seems as if they did so almost completely, keeping the pregnant woman as ignorant as possible and allowing her to participate as little as possible. In 1937 Dr. Roy Finney described the modern birth experience:

> Arriving [at the hospital], she is immediately given the benefit of one of the modern analgesics or pain-killers. Soon she is in a dreamy, half-conscious state at the height of a pain, sound asleep between spasms. Though hours must elapse before the infant appears, her conscious self is through; the rest is up to the doctor and her own reflexes.
>
> She knows nothing about being taken to a spotlessly clean delivery room, placed on a sterile table, draped with sterile sheets; neither does she see her attendants, the doctor and the nurses, garbed for her protection in sterile white gowns and gloves; nor the shiny boiled instruments and antiseptic solutions. She does not hear the cry of her baby when first he feels the chill of this cold world, or see the care with which the doctor repairs such lacerations as may have occurred. She is, as most of us want to be when severe pain has us in its grasp—asleep. Finally she awakens in smiles, a mother with no recollection of having become one. [6–7]

Although this is no longer the prevalent attitude, there are yet some male doctors who would rather conduct a delivery this way.

Over the last few centuries, as male and female midwives and doctors struggled for control in the delivery room, the mother (or mother-to-be) had less and less control over and less and less knowledge of what was happening to her and her as yet unborn child. Add to this situation the high rate of infant mortality, the incidence of childbed fever, and other problems, and the intellectual-emotional climate is ripe for folk belief; from folk beliefs about why this baby has a strange birthmark or that baby was stillborn, to folk beliefs which attempt to explain why this baby's complexion is not like anyone else's in the family or that baby grew up to be "bad." And these beliefs, or beliefs like them, continue to exist—even among women who have had childbirth education courses.

In fact, the July 1980 issue of *American Baby* included an article entitled "Pregnancy: Fact or Fiction" which presented a pregnancy quiz.

True/False Questions:

1. If a pregnant woman raises her arms above her head, the umbilical cord will wrap around the baby's neck.
2. If a pregnant woman swims or bathes, the baby may drown.
3. By smoking one cigarette a day, the pregnant woman may lower the baby's birthweight.
4. If an expectant mother suffers a severe fright, her child may inherit the fear.
5. Tea and cocoa can have adverse effects on the disposition of the unborn child.
6. Wine is good for pregnant women because it thickens the blood.
7. A woman loses a tooth for each pregnancy.
8. The baby's sex can be determined by the way a pregnant woman carries the baby.
9. The blood of the pregnant woman flows through the baby's blood to provide oxygen and nourishment.
10. A pregnant woman needs 2,000–3,000 calories daily and should gain at least 23 pounds. (Jimenez 54, 56)

Six of the ten items in the quiz (numbers 1, 2, 4, 6, 7, and 8) are based directly on common folk beliefs; four of the items (numbers 1, 2, 4, and 8) also appear in the collection on which this study is based.

The serious tone of the article surrounding the quiz suggests that the purpose of the article or quiz may have been to correct medical misinformation of which the readers might be possessed. *American Baby*'s mailing list comes from maternity shops, infant supply shops, and obstetricians; the magazine obviously pays for itself by selling advertising as it is sent to the expectant or new mother free of charge. It must, therefore, be directed largely at women in the middle and upper classes, women who—generally speaking—would want to learn more about pregnancy and childbirth and who would also be able to pay for the advertised products. *American Baby*'s publication of this article suggests that many of these women do have folk beliefs about pregnancy, and materials collected for this study support that view as well.

The folk beliefs collected in this project share certain characteristics. First, of the more than 300 women interviewed, this study concentrates on the 58 who attended some form of childbirth education class to receive instruction in addition to that given by their doctors. Most of those classes were in the Lamaze technique. Second, all of the 58 women had had children recently, most within the last five years. Third, most admitted to observing some folk belief. Only 8 of the 58 women interviewed maintained that they had observed no traditional practices whatever. (As will be discussed later, many said that they followed certain traditional practices—but not because they believed in them.) Fourth, the women interviewed lived within the same geographical area, Pitt County and surrounding counties in eastern North Carolina, an area which not only has a medical school and active childbirth education groups, but also has outreach programs in the county health offices and nurse-midwives practicing out of at least one obstetrician's office. Finally, most of the women interviewed seem to have had about the same amount of formal education and seem to have been from the same middle-class or above socioeconomic group.

A total of 133 beliefs was collected from the 58 female informants (see appendix). The beliefs fall into seven major categories: ways of determining the sex of an unborn child; factors which will mark the child; factors which can influence the health of the child; ways of inducing labor; factors contributing to the well-being of the mother; factors which affect the psychological character of the child; and miscellaneous. The separate beliefs and the number of times each belief appears have also been listed. There were 45 separate beliefs shared among 50 women; 8 women maintained that they had no traditional beliefs and followed no traditional practices.

The most popular category includes various ways for determining the sex of an unborn child. This category contains the most separate beliefs (10), the highest number of incidents (54), and the most popular single belief: the sex of an unborn child can be determined by the way in which the mother carries the child within her body. Generally, the informants said that if the baby is carried high it is a girl and if it is carried low it is a boy; but, of course, there were a few variants maintaining the opposite. That belief occurs 21 times and accounts for 15.8 percent of the total 133 incidents. The second most popular belief in this category (and tied for second overall), that a suspended ring or nail will indicate the sex of the fetus by its movement, occurs 14 times. The other 8 beliefs in this category contain a total of 19 incidents among them. The total number of incidents in this category, 54, is 40.6 percent of the total 133 incidents; and the total number of beliefs, 10, is 22.2 percent of the total 45.

The second most popular category, the factors which can physically mark a baby, contains 8 separate beliefs and 30 total incidents—the second highest occurrence of beliefs and incidents, but a significant drop in the number of incidents from Category 1. The most popular belief in this second category, that a mother who touches herself after a fright will mark a baby, occurs 10 times. The other 7 beliefs contain a total of 20 incidents. The 8 separate beliefs in this category are 17.7 percent of the total 45; and the 30 incidents are 22.5 percent of the total 133.

The third category, those factors which can affect the health of the baby, is the last large category. It contains 7 beliefs and 24 incidents; but it would be a very small category save for its most popular belief: Reaching up over your head while pregnant can cause the baby to strangle in its own umbilical cord. This belief occurs 14 times—10.5 percent of the total 133 incidents. Among the remaining 6 beliefs in this category, and all of the other beliefs occurring in the other 4 categories, 1 occurs 4 times, 2 occur 3 times, 2 occur 2 times, and the remaining 21 occur only 1 time each.

It is not surprising that there are so many beliefs about determining the sex of an unborn child. For many reasons, people have wanted to know the sex of their offspring as quickly as possible, and medical science has only recently been able to accommodate this desire before the actual birth. In the rather long interim, various methods of predicting the unborn child's sex were developed, and many of these methods are still in use today—some are even practiced by childbirth education instructors and by nurses in Pitt County Memorial Hospital's obstetrics section. It must be noted here, however, that a woman who tries one or more of these methods often says that she did it "just for fun" at a baby shower or other such event. There are others, though, who do believe seriously in one or more of these methods and usually know someone, occasionally a nurse or childbirth education instructor, who has an 85 to 95 percent accuracy in such predictions.

Categories 2 and 3—factors which will mark a baby and factors which will influence the health or disposition of the baby—may be a bit harder to account for. Both may have been triggered originally by a guilt reflex on the part of the mothers who, not knowing the reasons for their babies' unusual characteristics, had to have some external rationale. These women needed some assurance that their children's abnormalities were not the fault of the pregnant women but rather caused by some external agency. This would be especially true among people who believe that God shows his judgments through phenomenological portents. The popularity of such beliefs in eastern North Carolina may well be the result of the highly traditional nature of the area. Fundamentalist religions have a strong hold there, and families—of all socioeconomic classes—tend to be very close. A pregnant woman's aunt, grandmother, or mother could be a powerful force in requiring her to adhere to certain "old timey" ways, in spite of other, more modern attitudes. This same analysis would hold true for Category 5, factors contributing to the well-being of the mother, Category 6, factors which affect the psychological character of the child, and Category 7, miscellaneous.

Category 4, the various methods of inducing labor, deserves some special mention in spite of its relatively small size. The beliefs about bumpy roads or heavy work (especially moving furniture or scrubbing floors) causing the onset of labor can be misleading. Some of these tasks, like getting the baby's room ready, are often done at the last minute, while others are usually employed only when the mother-to-be is already a week or more past her "due date." In such instances, these measures—and similar ones such as sitting on a washing machine or taking a laxative—might well be effective. Today, these beliefs might appear infrequently for two reasons. On the one hand, more physicians are willing to induce labor artificially; and on the other, more Lamaze and other childbirth education mothers are willing to let labor begin when it will.

Overall, the popularity of Category 1—contrasted to the popularity of Categories 2 through 7—suggests that as medical information is disseminated to pregnant women their beliefs based on erroneous medical suppositions decrease. Other studies, both formal and informal, in eastern North Carolina indicated that among women who have had no childbirth education courses beliefs based on erroneous medical suppositions are plentiful. In fact, among these women—or among the population in general—such beliefs are even more numerous than are beliefs about determining the sex of the unborn child. This analysis is also supported by local childbirth education instructors who admit that the easiest beliefs to talk women out of are those which can easily be shown to be medically erroneous (Collins).

This is not meant to suggest that all folk beliefs are based on misinformation and are therefore wrong, foolish, or dangerous. There are folk beliefs in this collection which stand in contradiction to medical fact, but none of them (with the possible exception of eating corn starch to make the baby strong, Category 3, item F; or using a laxative to induce labor, Category 4, item D) is dangerous to the mother or the baby. And there are some folk beliefs, like walking a mile a day to keep the doctor away (Category 5, item D), which would be good for a pregnant woman; while others, like many of the ways of inducing labor (Category 4), might well be effective. Moreover, it should be noted that many of the women who practice these beliefs are educated people. Their beliefs are not the refuge of the ignorant; these beliefs do, in fact, coexist comfortably with some of the most recent knowledge concerning pregnancy and childbirth.

The materials collected for this study indicated that traditional beliefs are still held by many women who have had childbirth education courses, and it suggests that these women are more likely to practice one kind of belief than any other—although others were certainly represented in this collection. Such conclusions are limited to this group of informants, or perhaps a similar group, because these informants are a specific segment of the population of currently or recently pregnant women. Although such statistics were not rigorously kept, the 58 informants studied for this project were predominantly white, predominantly middle class or above (socially as well as economically), and predominantly positively disposed toward formal education and toward learning in a classroom setting.

It is interesting to note in this regard that the county health departments' outreach programs in eastern North Carolina are successfully dealing with poorer women, especially lower income and rural women, by educating them on a one-to-one basis, in cooperation with the local granny-midwives, or by teaching them in other than classroom settings (Stropnicky). These situations, which should be studied further in terms of the impact of these outreach programs on traditional beliefs, suggest that the materials which were the basis for this study are even more parochial than intended as they cover only the most visible of the childbirth education programs and their effects on traditional beliefs.

Appendix

Listed below are the seven general categories into which the beliefs collected for this study can be grouped. There are 45 distinct and separate items; repetition of specific beliefs brings the total number of incidents to 133. The number of beliefs and incidents is listed for each category, and the approximate percentage of the total is indicated.

1. Indicators of an unborn child's sex (10 beliefs/22.2 percent; 54 incidents/40.6 percent)
   - A. Where/how the fetus is carried (21/15.8 percent)
   - B. Suspending a ring/nail on a string/hair (14/10.5 percent)
   - C. Urine and drano color test (6/4.5 percent)
   - D. Fetal heart rate (5/3.8 percent)
   - E. Amount of fetal movement (3/2.2 percent)
   - F. Mother's dreams (1/0.75 percent)
   - G. Mother's cravings: sweet for girls, sour for boys (1/0.75 percent)
   - H. Mother's cravings: bananas for boys (1/0.75 percent)
   - I. Mother's complexion (1/0.75 percent)
   - J. Mother's indigestion (1/0.75 percent)

2. Factors which can physically mark an unborn child (8 beliefs/17.7 percent; 30 incidents/22.5 percent)
   - A. Severe fright (10/7.5 percent)
   - B. Food—especially strawberries (8/6.0 percent)
   - C. Heartburn (5/3.8 percent)
   - D. Laughing at someone (2/1.5 percent)
   - E. Looking at an ugly person (2/1.5 percent)
   - F. Beauty salon permanent (1/0.75 percent)
   - G. Rubbing someone's face (1/0.75 percent)
   - H. Looking at a fire (1/0.75 percent)

3. Factors affecting an unborn child's health (7 beliefs/15.5 percent; 24 incidents/18.0 percent)
   - A. Reaching up will cause unborn child to strangle (14/10.5 percent)
   - B. Looking at graves causes a stillbirth (4/3.0 percent)
   - C. Swimming can drown unborn baby (2/1.5 percent)
   - D. Hiccoughs mean unborn baby is growing (1/0.75 percent)
   - E. Copper bracelet keeps unborn baby healthy (1/0.75 percent)
   - F. Corn starch gives unborn baby strength (1/0.75 percent)
   - G. Rabbit on path: baby will hop, not crawl (1/0.75 percent)

4. Ways to induce labor (5 beliefs/11.1 percent; 9 incidents/6.8 percent)
   - A. Ride over a bumpy road (3/2.2 percent)
   - B. Do heavy work (3/2.2 percent)
   - C. Use a laxative (1/0.75 percent)
   - D. Sit on a washing machine (1/0.75 percent)
   - E. Drive a car at normal menstrual time (1/0.75 percent)

5. Factors which affect the welfare, health, or comfort of the mother (7 beliefs/15.5 percent; 8 incidents/6.0 percent)

   A. No sex during the last month of pregnancy (2/1.5 percent)
   B. Knife under bed cuts labor pain (1/0.75 percent)
   C. Kill a snake and baby will breech (1/0.75 percent)*
   D. Walk a mile a day to keep the doctor away (1/0.75 percent)
   E. Sleep on all sides for good circulation (1/0.75 percent)
   F. Do not be around paint (1/0.75 percent)
   G. Stay away from strong chemicals/cleaners (1/0.75 percent)

   *This item could also be included in Category 3, but it was reported by the informant as something she was aware of for her own health.

6. Factors which affect/indicate an unborn child's psychological character (4 beliefs/8.9 percent; 4 incidents/3.0 percent)

   A. Drink and the baby will crave liquor (1/0.75 percent)
   B. Mother's disposition affects the child (1/0.75 percent)
   C. Listen to music; child will be musical (1/0.75 percent)
   D. Mother's finger in a pickle jar turns pickles white during first trimester, child will be evil (1/0.75 percent)

7. Miscellaneous (4 beliefs/8.9 percent; 4 incidents/3.0 percent)

   A. To have a girl, use white vinegar douche (1/0.75 percent)
   B. Death is near three times during labor (1/0.75 percent)
   C. Do not set up nursery until after child is born (1/0.75 percent)
   D. Do not comb anyone else's hair while pregnant (1/0.75 percent)

References

Collins, Arlene, CBE Instructor. Interview. October 6, 1980.

Cutter, Irving, and Henry Viets. *A Short History of Midwifery.* Philadelphia: Saunders, 1964. This volume is an updated version of Cutter's 1934 publication of the same title; the additional materials were added by Viets.

Donegan, Jane B. *Women and Men Midwives: Medicine, Morality, and Misogyny in Early America.* Westport, Conn.: Greenwood, 1978.

Donnison, Jean. *Midwives and Medical Men: A History of Inter-Professional Rivalries and Women's Rights.* New York: Schocken, 1977.

Finney, Roy. *The Story of Motherhood.* New York: Liveright, 1937.

Jimenez, Sherry Lynn Mims. "Pregnancy: Fact or Fiction." *American Baby* (July 1980): 54, 56.

Stropnicky, Elizabeth, OB/GYN. Interview. October 9, 1980.

Thoms, Herbert. *Our Obstetrics Heritage of a Safe Childbirth.* Hamden, Conn.: Shoe String, 1960.

10. Aesthetic Agency in the Folk Medical Practices and Remembrances of North Carolinians

Karen Baldwin

Scientifically demonstrable efficacy and/or invested belief, issues of extreme importance to the study of *any* system of medicine, are not the only measures of relevance for maintenance of folk medical information and practice. Besides historical, social, and psychological functions served by the body of health-medical knowledge within a group, there are also aesthetic currents of preference for folk medicine which support its continued use or at least remembrance—measures of form, imagery, metaphor, and culturally appropriate performance. My interest here is in the effective artistry, the metaphoric resonances, the structured forms of expressive performance by which folk medical knowledge is normally transmitted.

The research materials I have drawn on are from my own fieldwork and from that of supervised student collectors who interviewed family and community members, as well as healer-specialists and their patients, and submitted their work to the East Carolina University Folklore Archive. The students' documentation of living traditions comprises both fairly brief statements of folk medical ideas and practice, what they and their informants understand as "beliefs" or "cures" or "remedies," and more extended narratives of personal experiences involving folk medicine as a function of family or community life.

First, I discuss how this corpus of statements and narratives simultaneously displays a variety of attitudes about folk medicine, revealing tenets of both belief and disbelief within a given region or ethnic group. Then I suggest possibilities for interpreting folk medical expressive forms, employing a scheme by which aesthetically evaluated entities are understood to be symbolic; expressive of cultural, group, or even individual values; artistically structured and patterned; and understood to have a source recognized as authoritative. I propose that there is aesthetic agency which can be significant to the retention, recreation, currency, and future of folk medical knowledge and practice.

North Carolinians from all stations of life and regions of the state, from the Appalachians to the Outer Banks barrier islands, have been reporting their home remedies and health beliefs, along with many other kinds of folk traditions, to ECU American Folklore students for twenty years. The students have collected narratives and songs, recipes, crafts, occupational traditions, childlore, architectural traditions, customary behaviors, and much more, from "exotic others," as well as within their own kin groups and communities. The health and medical beliefs and practices these students documented through the years, then, constitute only a portion of the archive's total holdings. That portion is significant, though. Among the archive's 5,000 manuscripts and 50,000 discrete items, there are some 800 manuscripts and 7,500 individually recorded items of health-medical belief and practice.

It is a stunning amount of material, which, in overview, importantly demonstrates the repetition and subtle variations characterizing folk cultural forms, the elements of major contrast among diverse ethno-regional cultures, the dynamics affecting folk traditional modes of expression by which change occurs, and the integral place health-medical beliefs and practices hold in folk cultural systems of scientific knowledge, technology, and art. Indeed, folklore archives are best able to display the broadest scope and the most articulate vitality of tradition in any region of the country where they exist. They are invaluable resources for folklorists and anthropologists, social and art historians. Folklore archives are, in addition, invaluable for clinical medical professionals, because in their collections are recorded attitudes and practices on which individuals depend for health maintenance, self-diagnosis, and home treatment of a variety of physiologically and psychologically disordering conditions—attitudes and practices which affect individuals' interactions with the clinical medical community, but are not likely to be offered as background by patients presenting themselves for treatment in clinical settings.

The North Carolina materials which inform and illustrate my argument here demonstrate both active practice and active remembrance of folk medical knowledge among a wide social range of individuals and groups of Carolina folks, not just Watauga County mountaineers or Harker's Island mariners. A majority of the materials are reported as vestiges of an older, less technologically infiltrated society, and reflect the bias that, once persons have access to "advanced" knowledge and clinical arenas, they will supplant their home self-treatments with what the scientific tradition offers; the old cures and information about their use will die.

The fact is that information about the old cures, whether magic or herbal, exists in tradition, even when active practice is no longer recognized as appropriate. Grandmother's remedy for earache using warm hog urine or sweet oil exists as traditional knowledge in generations beyond grandmother. Her remedy may still be acted upon, or, just as significantly, it may be valued as part of the family's remembrance of her and be a medium of narrated information exchange through which the grandmother is orally, traditionally memorialized. Folk remedies are also being recreated, incorporating agents only recently available. People apply WD-40 to arthritic stiff joints and spray starch for the irritation of chicken pox, and urinate into a pile of Drāno in the backyard for pregnancy testing. The old cures are not dying and new cures are being developed. Why?

One answer which regularly turns up in informant explanations of their use for home remedy agents is that many are, indeed, efficacious. But folk medical ideas and prescriptions are not maintained simply because they "work" in scientific terms. There is also a complex of aesthetic features at work with folk medical statements, experience narratives, and enactments. Artistic patterning, symbolic meaning, cultural value, and authoritative source exert what can be a tremendous influence on the continued use or, at least, remembrance of folk medical information. There is a magic of metaphoric resonance, which helps make symbolic sense of the cures for the tradition bearers, structured by artistic features, coupled with or arising from having the cure knowledge transmitted by or received from the proper source—this aesthetic complex, indeed, may be a partial reason why folk medical information systems are still so healthy, so actively practiced.

This focus on the aesthetic agency of folk medical information and enactment does not deny the importance of understood or proven efficacy, nor can the issue of invested belief be entirely set aside. The archive materials express a significant range of attitudes—from esoterically held belief to exoterically differentiating disbelief (Hufford 1982). Indeed, one service a broad survey of folk medical materials can provide, perhaps better than in-depth, contextually based studies, is a clear view of the coexistence of both belief and disbelief traditions within the same cultural groups. In order to responsibly address the corpus of folk medical materials such as exist in folklore archives, one must permit that any such collection will demonstrate both what is believed and what is disbelieved, what is understood to be efficacious and what is well known not to work, what belongs to cultural groups and what falls outside the cultural ken of those groups.

One set of mainstream notions revealed in the ECU materials regards folk medicine as quaintly irrelevant, if not as superstition-bound hazards to health. Concomitantly, archive reports reveal preferences for what is recognized within families and communities as home remedies or "old timey cures," preferences based in overtly expressed ideas about financial economy, historical relevance (that is, standing the test of time), preferences for natural, familiar agents (or at least those with pronounceable names), and personal or social appropriateness (that is, the significance of source for active remembrance or performance of remedies and medical advices). Both sets of ideas occur in archive holdings and sometimes they coexist in tension with each other. Whether they express belief or disbelief, though, the prescriptive statements, experience narratives, or descriptions of enactments indicate a complex of aesthetic agency in their continued use or remembrance.

The prescriptive statement is definitely one form in which the information about a condition and its amelioration is transmitted. Succinctness and implied objectivity are regular features of the prescription, regardless of the agents mentioned:

> A good remedy for morning sickness is two tablespoons of salt and milk.
>
> [Compare Brown 1775 for "liver trouble"][1] Take a handful of bark from a cucumber tree. Cut in pieces about the size of a dime and fill a pint whiskey bottle. Then fill bottle with corn whiskey. Leave to soak for 3 days. Then pour whiskey off of bark. Take 1 tsp. before each meal and at bedtime for arthritis.

Cause-effect and declarative structures, often invoking sympathetic, magical similitive analogy or startlingly descriptive, perhaps playful imagery, infrequently employing poetic-mnemonic devices of rhyme and meter—all are elements of the artistry and the affect of such as the following:

> If you are four months pregnant and can walk up a staircase backwards while drinking a martini, then you will miscarry.
>
> If you are pregnant and accept an article (crib, toy) from the mother of a baby who recently died (then) something will be wrong with your child.
>
> Feed a cold and starve a fever.

And, indeed, the same forms and artistic patterns are capable of transmitting content which is credibly esoteric as well as content which is strange; content which expresses exoteric disbelief in the "weird" ideas and practices of "exotic" others. "If you want to get rid of someone, just put some of their hair in a jar and throw it in a ditch. That person will soon die." (Reported from a twenty-two-year-old, white, Beaufort County woman who reports she heard this from some of her black pupils in Martin County.) Cultural dissonance may be experienced much closer to home when a younger person confronts the "old-fashioned" ideas of a folk group elder. "[Compare Brown 2032] If you want to make your arthritis better you should drink a teaspoon of salt water each day." (Reported from a seventy-six-year-old, white, Dare County woman, by her college student granddaughter. The collector adds: "I don't know where Grandmother got this idea but she used to have us bring her a jar of sea water when her arthritis was acting up. Had to come from the ocean, too, not just salt water from the sound.")

Parodizing familiar traditions underscores their significance. Like the students' parody of the *Battle Hymn of the Republic*—"Mine eyes have seen the glory of the burning of the school / We have tortured every teacher, we have broken every rule"—folk medicine parodies "break the rules" of authority in health belief systems in order to mend them whole again with humor. Their evocative imagery and feigned objectivity make these parody examples work very well as chiding perversions of cold cure practices.

> If you think you're getting a cold, you should get in bed, and put a hat on one of the bedposts. Then you lay in bed and drink whiskey until you see two hats. And when you sober up, you don't have the cold any more.

> The way to cure a cold is to buy a box of aspirin and a pint of liquor. Go home, get ready for bed, throw the aspirin out the window and drink the pint. Next morning the cold will be gone.

> Best thing for a cold . . . is to undress and stand in front of an open window and catch pneumonia and then them doctors could do something for that!

However formulaically structured, metaphorically resonant, and artful brief statements of health and medical belief and practice might be, when they are reported merely as texts, dislodged from their enabling, appropriate contexts, they easily can be viewed as faintly comic curiosities or exemplary dangers of ignorance. The notions of irrelevance and potential harm persist, supported, in good measure, by repeated publication of folk medicine materials almost exclusively as lists of prescriptive verbal capsules of what to use and how to use it, albeit sometimes made more palatable by the poetic assonance of "An apple a day keeps the doctor away." The vigorously legalistic disclaimer with which Jack and Olivia Solomon introduce the "Asfidity" section of their *Cracklin Bread and Asfidity,* a collection for a general audience edited from the student-collected archive materials at the University of Alabama, tells my point well. "The editors do not recommend that you experiment with the folk remedies that follow, however, [*sic*] sensible they may appear. They are presented as folklore, not as serious medicine. *We issue a clear, definite warning against these prescriptions.* If you happen to use them already, that is your business. Even if you do, consult your physician, not us or the contributors" (1979, 128).

The tenor of such a warning is startling, given its place in what is otherwise a paean to the nobility and ingenuity of Alabama country folks. But the subtextual message is clear. The curative and preventative statements are plainly (and, therefore, *dangerously*) set forth without any reference to the more complex information necessary for their use, and without any cultural or community background information, save the names of the persons from whom they were collected. This sort of culturally "desensitized" list presentation of cure and belief statements is possible because of the editors' reinforcement of the well-entrenched notion of folk medicine as distinct from "serious" or "real" medicine.

Academic treatments of the same kinds of herbal and magic cure statements need no such warnings. The scholarly apparatus of Hand's explication and two-volume edition, *Popular Beliefs and Superstitions from*

North Carolina, Volumes 6 and 7 of *The Frank C. Brown Collection of North Carolina Folklore,* precludes the reader's mistaking the more than 2,700 comprehensively annotated items of health and curative belief as self-treatment alternatives to "serious" medicine. But popular collections, such as the Solomons offer, and scholarly treatments, such as Hand's, depend on an understanding of folk medicine as a corpus of texts—verbal formulations capable of abstraction from their cultural contexts. This has both helped and hindered the study of folk medicine.

For much of the history of the discipline, folklorists have concerned themselves with a generic analytical approach to fieldwork and to reporting their collectanea in print or organizing it in research archives. Traditionally, then, health and medical beliefs—like quilts, tales, dances, and recipes—have been regarded as products, at some point separable from community and individual cultural contexts. Scholars concerned with understanding the cultural symbols and the metaphors of magic embedded in folk beliefs have used essentially literary approaches to medical and health statements, as well as to folktale, balladry, and proverb forms.

In addition, folklorists have tended to collect and concentrate their textual analyses on folk cures which require bases in magic or faith-derived belief systems. Strictly herbal-naturopathic cures more often have been treated as folk pharmacology, more the province of ethnobotonists than folklorists, based on the empirical observations and oral, traditionally maintained reports of cause-effect relationships from practitioners whose training and expertise is community based and folk cultural.

The textual approach allows for broad surveys of materials and the cultural differentiation of ideas, but as Hufford further suggests in his recent essay, "Folk Healers," the generic approach presents problems for the study of folk health belief *systems.*

> Folk medicine and its practitioners have never really found a comfortable or consistent place in the generic organizational scheme that has characterized folklore scholarship since its inception. Most often in American folklore studies folk medicine has been considered a subdivision of the "minor genre" called superstition (a term now generally avoided because of its pejorative connotations) or folk belief. Since the general concept is derived from the study of literature it naturally leads one to think in terms of discrete products of language such as poems or novels. Consequently, the study of folk healing began with the collection and listing of cures and "beliefs" [as texts]. (306)

One outcome of this generic way of thinking has been the reporting of information primarily in abbreviated forms. Such an approach benefits the documentation of quantities of materials and supports cross-culturally comparative and historical studies of their content. As Hufford agrees, "some very useful scholarship dealing with questions of origin and geographical distribution has resulted from this enumerative method" (1983, 306).

Archives hold and reflect the variety and artistry of such statements from the communities whose traditions they represent, and these are intrinsically interesting, extrinsically evocative. Especially because cure and health belief statements are usually presented without significant explanation and reported without meaningful contextual description, they are in several ways very much like biomedical physicians' prescriptions. Their often proverb-like sententious form is meant to reinforce their palliative effect. When the source for the advice is unknown or not recognized as authoritative, though, the use of the prescription, whether folk culturally based or from biomedicine, is understood as potentially dangerous. Both the biomedical and the folk traditional prescription require appropriate context for their best outcome. When folk health and medical advices are appropriately situated, they are embedded in and draw significant meaning simultaneously from all aspects of their natural surroundings, including the personnel, the performance, the physical environment, the social and chronological time, and the dynamic-conservatory tenets of the cultural tradition.

The personal experience narration, the evidentiary anecdote, is a primary means of communicating information and managing effect for any health maintenance and curative system, folk or not. We tell what one elder calls "organ recitals" about our surgeries (Hufford, Hunt, Zeitlin 32). Women exchange gyno-narratives and mothers deliver labor and childbirth sagas in their postpartum experience tellings. Construction workers inform each other, through on-the-job injury stories, about the first-aid applications of sawdust for cuts and lubricating oil for minor burns. Secretaries and store clerks tell about the application of sewing machine oil for the head congestion of a cold.

> [Compare Brown 1126] You know that old woman in here a while ago that bought those three dresses? She told me if I would take some number 1 machine oil, and put it on my face like this (running her finger down her nose and out over her cheeks and finally across her

> top lip), she said my head would clear right up. In an hour's time, she said, I would be able to tell the difference. You know, I'm going to try it. (Reported from a 29-year-old black Hertford County woman. Collector adds: "I worked with the informant in a store during the Christmas holidays. We both had very bad head colds.")

Family members, too, transmit their experiences with folk medicine as well as with physician's medicine through the personal narrative.

> My daddy was cured of a cancer by a home remedy. He had cancer on his hand and the doctor said not to let anyone mess with it. There was this family in Onslow County who had a concoction of herbs that had been handed down from one generation to another. So Papa went up there and they put the formula on his hand. The doctor had said that he wouldn't have Papa's hand for the world. But that formula healed his hand. I saw it and it's the truth. (Reported from a 60-year-old white New Hanover County woman.)

The first part of the attraction, the magic, of the folk medicine aesthetic is a matter of source. Assessments of authority for systems of knowledge and practice influence our judgments in folk traditional contexts as well as in clinical, scientific contexts. I offer one of my own experience narratives as illustration.

One day in the English Department office I was startled to a stop by a senior colleague who asked if I knew someone who could "talk off" warts. "Well, yes," I replied, slowly, wondering what was behind his request. The colleague explained. His daughter was having trouble with growths on her hands, and their dermatologist had suggested a folk healer might be an appropriate source of help.

Indeed, I knew of a farmer near Blackjack with whom I'd talked one evening in his home about how his kinswoman transmitted power to "carry off" both human and bovine warts with whispered words, and, in that same moment, I could think of one of my students who reported that his father, a supermarket manager in nearby Wilson County, was regularly visited at the store by patients seeking the same help. I had no qualms about telling him the name of the farmer, nor did I regard his request as untoward.

Despite his Anglo, middle-class, educated background, or perhaps because of it, this colleague had every good cultural reason to approach me for such information. He is a native of the area, and probably knew about "wart talkers" in his early years, certainly much sooner than I, an "outsider" from Philadelphia. But within his family and round of personal associates there might predictably be no other, no more authoritative, source for the name of a wart healer than the transmigrated Yankee director of the Folklore Archive.

I was cautiously curious about the suggestion having come from a physician, though. As it turned out, the person my colleague named is a medical professional who is known to be sensitive to the folk healing traditions in this region, and, sometimes, will include mention of those as options for patients. I passed along the farmer's name. The daughter, I heard later, opted for a clinical procedure, and all was well with her warts. The experience was, for me, a telling example of the history and future of folk medical practices, illustrating the role of folk medicine in the present lives of one family of North Carolinians.

Disquieting as it may be to some, among my American Folklore students there are always a number of folk traditional responses to the question: "What do you do to get rid of warts?" The folk-cured students have rubbed their warts with a stolen dishrag or the flesh of a freshly cut "Irish" (never "sweet") potato (Brown 2543–49), then buried the potato slice at midnight or the dishrag under the front porch (2578–2612) and waited for the warts to disappear. Some have applied extruded dandelion juice (2522). Not unusually, one among them will have had warts "talked off" (2690, 2695–96, 2701) or have heard of another whose warts were "bought" (2675–84) by a hometown person with some "gift" for wart removal.

The rationalists, and those culturally naive about such ideas, easily scoff at the notion that warts could go away with words, or for the price of a penny, but they are rapt by such discussion as transpired one day when an African-American woman volunteered her grandmother's Bible verse cure for a nosebleed: three rapid repetitions of Ezekiel 16:6 (882).

I pressed the woman to explain the circumstances of her knowledge of her grandmother's cure. It turns out that it was the student's own nosebleed which happened during a visit to her grandmother's house that occasioned the cure. The woman explained in detail what she did and how she felt. Her own rational conclusion was that she was so "scared," so moved by the power of everything which came to bear at that moment—her own faithful background in the church, awareness of her grandmother's strong faith, respect for her grandmother's authority, reverence for the text she was told to read, and anxiety to effect the cure properly—

that, not only did the bleeding stop, but, as she shrugged her shoulders to admit, she *believed,* then, that the Bible verse cure had much to do with "stopping the blood." At the same time, she agreed that her emotional state undoubtedly had the effect of constricting capillary circulation, but because she had been able to remember vividly, and with such culturally significant resonance, that first occasion for cure with the prescribed repetition of the Biblical word "blood," she said she would use that cure again. Why? Because, she said, "it *works.*"

The young woman's surface meaning, so simply stated, easily could be understood by all who heard her story: "The bleeding stopped." There are further implications of aesthetic agency, though, which include much more than simply the desired outcome, and with which she was much too culturally familiar to be able to articulate in a classroom environment. What worked was a whole complex of cultural features necessary to the procedure, including family connection and social structure, belief in the healing effects of religious faith, with the underlying homeopathic sympathy of three repetitions of the word which names and controls the condition.

Harry Crews, the novelist, invokes the efficacious power of the healer who names and controls injury and pain in the story from his Georgia boyhood memory of having been catapulted off the end of a line of children playing "pop the whip" too close to the scalding vat at a family hog butchering. Only Crews's head was not submerged in water hot enough to boil the tough hairs off a hog or scald a child to death. First he was rushed to the doctor in whose treatment rooms he noticed that his skin peeled off when he touched it. Later, at home in bed, he was visited by Hollis Toomey, the "fire talker" from his home county. "He talked to the fire like an old and respected adversary," Crews wrote (116). "At some point while he talked he put his hands on me, one of them spread out big as a frying pan, and I was already as cool as spring water. But I had known I would be from the moment I had seen him standing in the door. . . . The tone of his voice made me know that he was locked in a real and terrible conflict with the fire" (117).

Crews's self-conscious artistry is recapitulated in the experience narrative collected by an ECU folklore student from a forty-three-year-old white woman burn healer near Farmville, who explains with precision about the linkages there must be between practitioner and patient, between generations in a group. The woman's initial expressions of disbelief about the power she was given artistically establish the authority she bears as healer. As she proceeds through the narration of an increasingly more integrated series of healing episodes—involving her infant daughter, her neighbor, a stranger referred by a neighbor, and herself, the total narrative, excerpted here, is transformed as a metaphor which speaks in gifted words about burn healing as a central, rather than a peripheral, tradition, one which, in essence, defines the relationship among the individual, her family, and community.

> Well, the beginning was . . . I have to go back to the beginning. When I was 12, my mother was teaching me how to fry chicken. Y'always pierce the liver before you fry it. And I was standing there at the stove and the liver exploded all up and down my arm and she called him [the teller's grandfather] and he came around there and talked the fire out of it . . . and I never had a blister; it never hurt . . . and I just knew I was ruined for life! He says it so low over the burn that you never hear what he says . . . and it just fascinated me. But that was my first real encounter with it . . . and I never thought about it any more 'til he got really, really bad off and was in the nursing home and I was pregnant with my daughter and he . . . I knew he was gonna' pass away before long and I went to see him. In fact, it was the last time I saw him . . . and I told him that I knew he didn't have anything to really leave, you know, material thing, but I wanted him to give me the secret of how to help people when they got burned. So he made my husband go out of the room and he told me what it was.
>
> I was really surprised because I thought it was really gonna be some big mumbo jumbo thing . . . some real mystical thing . . . and I came out of the room and I was just, I was just floored! I thought . . . this . . . you know, this is really weird, because, I thought, anybody could say this, you know, and do it. But he told me the real thing behind it was, you have to have a lot of faith. And the person [patient] has to have a lot of faith. They have to believe that you can do this thing for them, or it doesn't work. So I really didn't have a real occasion to use it until my oldest daughter was about 18 or 19 months old and we moved into our first house and we had a floor furnace—it was during the winter time and she walked across it and tripped and fell forward with both of her hands and knees. So I immediately picked her up and tried it. I thought, "What the heck! It won't hurt to try!" And it worked! And I was just so floored and flabbergasted, I just thought it was the greatest thing!

> Yeah, I guess my faith in it was so strong, that it just, it did it. In a few minutes, she quit crying. It never blistered up; she never had the first scar. It was just, I was just totally delighted, you know, that I had something that I could really use. And I told one of my best girl-friends about it . . . they lived on the other side of town . . . and she called me up one night, about two or three months after that and she had been cooking and she wanted to know if she got her husband to bring her around there, would I talk the fire out of it . . . and I said, "Sure, come on!" So they came around there and I talked the fire out of her. She had been cooking, and . . . you know how you're steaming stuff . . . and she'd lifted the pot lid and it just automatically, just blistered her, you know; it was fiery red. And a few minutes after she had come around there, and I had, you know, talked the fire out of it . . . it turned just as nice and white and it didn't burn any more. The color goes away and everything.
>
> I've even done it on myself—especially cooking. I was cooking something in there on the stove, and I went to pull the pan out of the oven and didn't have the lid on it and the water, it was just like scalding hot water, just splashed all over, up and down my wrist, on my hand, and it just . . . I just thought, "Jeez! Look at that! I'm gonna be ruined!" But I just did it to myself, and it's amazing to me how it does it. (ECU Folklore Archive)

When we consider the artistry of folk medical traditions as well as their science, the metaphors of meaning become as significant for maintenance of those health systems as scientific proofs of their efficacy. Mrs. Emma Dupree, an African-American herbalist from Fountain, speaks about her special knowledge, her plants, and her patients' well-being in images of wholeness and continuity. Hers is a faith-based tradition, as well as naturopathic, and she marks her sense of linkage with the tradition from the day of her birth, July 4, 1897.

> When I was born, I was the seventh one, the seventh sister. And they say the seventh one will be over-endowed in everything. . . . was born way back in the hard times—way back. We had no light, but we had a little bit in a lamp. And my daddy went for the doctor. . . . Meanwhile all of the oil from the lantern burnt out. And he hadn't gotten back by the time the oil burnt out. And my mother was in the dark. When he got back it had got day just like early in the morning. They had a

> glow—the yard, leaves, and the house glowed—and that light stayed until 10 in the day, and it was brighter than the sun when I was born. [My mother] says that's why I was so different. . . . People talked and I listened and my heart was big enough to hold all that. I talked different . . . was strong in my talking . . . I was just born to that. (Baldwin 50)

What Mrs. Dupree was "just born to" was a system of knowledge concerning the medicinal uses of the plant and other natural materials in her home area of Pitt County. As a young woman, she says, "I got to ramblin' that woods . . . got to makin' the woods my own," harvesting the plants she foraged in the sack she always had with her. She was also "just born to" a folk traditional sense of the natural environment in concert with the human community, and she often expresses this holistic view through comments which make similitive connections between the growth patterns of her house garden cultivated plants and the conformation of the human body. She held a maypop frond against her palm and said, "See, that looks near about like a man's hand." She severed the trunk root of a sweet flag plant, held it up by its feeder root "arms" and explained, "See, that grows near 'bout like a man does" (Baldwin 51–52).

Probably the most significant metaphoric construct she uses, though, is the idea of "labeling" her bottled preparations with her "mouth." Hers is an inescapably immediate, powerfully direct transmission of prescriptive uses for her "yerb" tonics and salves. She does not transmit anything in writing. She says, "I give the label with my mouth" (Baldwin 52).

There is, indeed, a high degree of interaction necessary between Mrs. Dupree and her patients, some of whom respectfully refer to her as "the doctor." She needs and accepts from them donations of the ingredients other than plant materials she uses, including honey, brown sugar, lemons, vinegar, and mineral water. Patients also provide many of the cleaned pickle and mayonnaise jars into which Mrs. Dupree decants her teas and tonics before dispensing them to patients received in her sitting room, just next to the kitchen where the preparations are made. There is no responsible way to segregate Mrs. Dupree's herbal knowledge or ameliorative products from the process of their production or the context of their administration. Mrs. Dupree knows that and, ultimately, so must all her patients. Her metaphors of wholeness and continuity, then, are direct expressions out of and indirect reflections from the actual circumstances of her knowledge and practice. They are, indeed, the most significant and encompassing elements of her herbal practice, the aesthetic agency of her enactments of herbal healing.

The ECU Folklore Archive materials demonstrate a rich tradition of active remembrance and continued practice which extends and reinterprets the traditional life of what some might consider dormant or dying folk medical ideas and expressive forms. There is good reason for a dermatologist and his middle-class, educated patient to consider the ministrations of a wart talker, good basis for the community existing among patients and practitioners of herbal medicine and faith-based burn healing. One can survey the members of extended kin communities in regions of the state and assemble the composite of home remedy knowledge and anecdotal evidence of practice there exists in prescriptive statements and cure recipes. One can discover the vitality of self health care and ameliorative practices in the causal structures of medical advice exchanged among coworkers describing the use of mass-manufactured, nonpharmaceutical agents. If scientific proof of efficacy or the necessity of invested belief were the only measures of relevance for such ideas and practices, the plethora of folk medical information held in folklore archives plausibly should not exist. There are other factors at work as well, empowering the knowers of folk medical ideas and practices and their family and community patients. My suggestion here is that some of the powerful resource of folk medical systems lies in the agency of the aesthetic realm. The aesthetic complex of symbolic, culturally expressive, structured, and patterned entities (statements, narratives, and enactments), emanating from authoritative sources and operating within intimately significant environments gives greater dimension to our understanding of the existence as well as the efficacy of contemporary folk medical practice and remembrance.

Notes

1. Bracketed numbers preceding or following archive texts indicate correspondence with materials listed in vol. 6 of *The Frank C. Brown Collection of North Carolina Folklore*, ed. Wayland D. Hand, *Popular Beliefs and Superstitions from North Carolina.* Those materials with no cross reference number have no correspondence with *Brown.*

References

Baldwin, Karen. "Mrs. Emma Dupree: 'That Little Medicine Thing.'" *North Carolina Folklore Journal* 32.2 (1984): 50–53.

Crews, Harry. *A Childhood: The Biography of a Place.* New York: Harper & Row, 1978.

Hand, Wayland D., ed. *Popular Beliefs and Superstitions from North Carolina.* Durham, N.C.: Duke University Press, 1961, 1964. Vols. 6, 7 of *The Frank C. Brown Collection of North Carolina Folklore.*

Hufford, David J. "Traditions of Disbelief." *New York Folklore* 3–4 (1982): 47–55.

———. "Folk Healers." *Handbook of American Folklore.* Ed. Richard M. Dorson. Bloomington: Indiana University Press, 1983.

Hufford, Mary, Marjorie Hunt, and Steven Zeitlin. *The Grand Generation: Memory, Mastery, Legacy.* Smithsonian Institution. Seattle: University of Washington Press, 1988.

Solomon, Jack, and Olivia Solomon. *Cracklin Bread and Asfidity.* Tuscaloosa: University of Alabama Press, 1979.

Bibliography

James Kirkland and

C. W. Sullivan III

An Exercise in Comprehensive Selection

While compiling this bibliography, we have often thought of the plight of the central character in Arnold van Gennep's "The Research Topic: Or, Folklore without End," which tells the story of a young scholar who began researching a single branch of folk tradition, the Evil Eye, at the age of eighteen and became so immersed in his work that he was still accumulating data at age fifty-four, by which time he had learned hundreds of languages, compiled 27,000 bibliography items, and written 12,000,000 notes. Unfortunately for the scholar, he died at his carrel in the Bibliothèque Nationale while updating his bibliography—without having published a single item.

Though our own efforts have been at once less ambitious and less traumatizing than those of van Gennep's scholar, we have been forced to wrestle with many of the same problems: the magnitude of the published record; the linguistic and cultural diversity of folk medical tradition bearers; the wide range of ethnographic, artistic, and scientific perspectives that have been brought to bear on this subject; and the constant publication of new studies that make any bibliography out of date as soon as it goes to press.

We have attempted to resolve these difficulties in two ways: first, by limiting our citations primarily to works in English; and second, by choosing from those works a representative cross section of books, chapters, and articles by folklorists, anthropologists, health care specialists, linguists, and other scholars from a variety of disciplinary perspectives. The result, we believe, is a selective but thorough reference work that documents not only the scholarship on the regional traditions discussed by the contributors to this book but also the extensive body of research devoted to other forms of folk medical belief and practice.

The selected bibliography which follows is, then, an attempt to supplement the works cited in the individual essays. As such, it has been limited to sources not cited elsewhere in the volume. Thus, the volume *Popular Beliefs and Superstitions* of *The Frank C. Brown Collection of North Carolina Folklore*—though obviously pertinent to bibliographic sections 1H and 3C—appears under neither heading because Kirkland, Croom, and Baldwin all cite it in their respective essays.

To facilitate access to these materials, we have organized this bibliography by topic. Section 1 identifies books and articles according to the traditional belief or practice named in the title and examined in the text. Section 2 does the same for practices more often considered a part of popular culture rather than folk or traditional culture. Sections 3–5 identify materials according to the geographic region in which they are found and tend to be studies that examine a broad range of traditional practices—medical and other. Sections 7–9 index general studies in medical folklore, medical anthropology, and medical sociology.

Because entries are not cross-referenced within the bibliography, readers should examine all pertinent categories. For example, someone seeking additional information on Native American shamans should look first in section 1 (Traditional Medical Beliefs and Practices), subsection B (Magic, Witchcraft, Shamanism, and Charms). The next step would be to examine section 4 (Ethnomedical Traditions in the United States), subsection A (Native American). Finally, the reader might turn to section 3 (American Folk Medicine: Regional Variation), under the appropriate geographical heading. Entries in sections 7–9 can be consulted for general background and additional context from disciplinary perspectives.

I. Traditional Medical Beliefs and Practices

A. Ethnobotany and Herbalism

Akimov, Iu. A., et al. "Antimicrobial Effect of Terpenes from savin *Juniperus sabina* L." *Biological Abstracts* 64.4 (1977): 3,051.

Allen-Wheeler, Jane. "A Herbalist's Shop in Honolulu: Traditional Merchandising in a Modern Setting." *Modern Material Culture: The Archaeology of Us*. Ed. Richard A. Gould and Michael B. Schiffer. New York: Academic, 1981. 101–12.

Altschul, Siri von Reis. *Drugs and Foods from Little-Known Plants: Notes in Harvard University Herbaria*. Cambridge, Mass.: Harvard University Press, 1973.

Anderson, Edward F. *Peyote: The Divine Cactus*. Tucson: University of Arizona Press, 1980.

Anonymous. "Remedies, Herb Doctors and Healers." *Foxfire 9*. Ed. Eliot Wigginton and Marjorie Bennett. Garden City, N.Y.: Anchor Press/Doubleday, 1985. 12–82.

Arena, J. M. *Poisoning: Toxicology, Symptoms, Treatments*. Springfield, Ill.: Thomas, 1974.

Ayensu, E. S. *Medicinal Plants of West Africa*. Algonac, Mich.: Reference, 1978.

Balls, Edward K. *Early Uses of California Plants*. Berkeley: University of California Press, 1962.

Barrois, Julie. "Herb Cures in an Isolated Black Community in the Florida Parishes." *Louisiana Folklore Miscellany* 3.1 (1970): 25–27.

Baskin, Esther. *The Poppy and Other Deadly Plants*. New York: Delacorte, 1967.

Beckett, Sarah. *Herbs for Clearing the Skin*. Wellingborough, Northamptonshire, England: Thorsons, 1973.

——. *Herbs for Prostate and Bladder Troubles*. Wellingborough, Northamptonshire, England: Thorsons, 1973.

Benoit, P. S., et al. "Biological and Phytochemical Evaluation of Plants." *Lloydia* 39 (1976): 160–71.

Body, A. P. "The Medical Plants of Berks County." *Pennsylvania Folklife* 18.1 (1968): 40–41.

Browner, C. H. "Criteria for Selecting Herbal Remedies." *Ethnology* 24.1 (1985): 13–32.

Carlson, Gustav G., and Volney H. Jones. "Some Notes on Uses of Plants by the Comanche Indians." *Papers of the Michigan Academy of Science, Arts, and Letters* 25 (1939): 526.

Chambliss, Charles E. "The Botany and History of Zizania Aquatica L. ('Wild Rice')." *Annual Report of the Smithsonian Institution* (1940): 369–82.

Chestnut, V. K. "Plants Used by the Indians of Mendocino County, California." *Contributions from the U.S. National Herbarium* 7.3. Washington, D.C.: GPO, 1902.

Clymer, R. Swinburne. *Nature's Healing Agents: The Medicines of Nature*. Quakertown, Penn.: Humanitarian Society, 1979.

Conway, David. *The Magic of Herbs*. New York: Dutton, 1973.

Core, E. L. "Ethnobotany of the Southern Appalachian Aborigines." *Economic Botany* 21 (1967): 198–214.

Corrigan, Desmond. "The Scientific Basis of Folk Medicine: The Irish Dimension." *Plant-Lore Studies*. Ed. Roy Vickery. London: Folklore Society, 1984. 10–42.

Coville, Frederick. "Notes on Plants Used by the Klamath Indians of Oregon." *Contributions from the U.S. National Herbarium* 5. Washington, D.C.: GPO, 1897–1901.

Crellin, John K., and Jane Philpott. Vol. 1: *Trying to Give Ease*; vol. 2: *A Reference Guide to Medicinal Plants*. Durham, N.C.: Duke University Press, 1990.

Cronquist, Arthur. *Asteraceae. Vascular Flora of the Southeastern United States*. Chapel Hill: University of North Carolina Press, 1980–90.

Croom, Edward M., Jr. "Documenting and Evaluating Herbal Remedies." *Economic Botany* 38.1 (1983): 13–27.

Curtain, L. S. M. *Healing Herbs of the Upper Rio Grande*. Santa Fe, N.M.: Rydal, 1947.

Densmore, F. "Uses of Plants by the Chippewa Indians." *Bureau of American Ethnology 44th Annual Report*. Washington, D.C.: Smithsonian, 1928.

Dimond, E. Grey. *More Than Herbs and Acupuncture*. New York: Norton, 1975.

Elmore, F. H. "Ethnobotany of the Navajo." *University of New Mexico Bulletin*. New York: AMS, 1978.

Elvin-Lewis, M. "Empirical Rationale for Teeth Cleaning Plant Selection." *Medical Anthropology* 3 (1979): 431–58.

Emboden, William A. *Narcotic Plants*. New York: Macmillan, 1972.

——. "Plant Hypnotics Among the North American Indians." *American Folk Medicine: A Symposium*. Ed. Wayland D. Hand. Berkeley: University of California Press, 1976. 159–69.

Evans, E. Raymond, Clive Kileff, and Karen Shelley. "That Was All We Ever Knew." *Herbal Medicine: A Living Force in the Appalachians*. Durham, N.C.: Duke University Medical Center, 1982.

Evans, J. P. "Medicinal Plants of the Cherokees." *Proceedings of the American Pharmaceutical Association* 8 (1859): 390–97.

Farnsworth, N. R., and G. A. Cordell. "A Review of Some Biologically Active Compounds Isolated from Plants as Reported in the 1974–75 Literature." *Lloydia* 39 (1976): 420–55.

Farnsworth, N. R., et al. "Potential Value of Plants as Sources of New Antifertility Agents." *Journal of Pharmaceutical Sciences* 64.4 (1975): 535–98.

Fernald, Merrit L., and Alfred C. Kinsey. *Edible Wild Plants of Eastern North America*. New York: Harper, 1958.

Fielder, Mildred. *Plant Medicine and Folklore*. New York: Winchester, 1975.

Fleisher, Mark S. "The Ethnobotany of the Clallam Indians of Western Washington." *Northwest Anthropological Research Notes* 14 (1980): 192–210.

Free, William Joseph. "A Note on Tobacco Magic." *North Carolina Folklore* 10.2 (1962): 9–10.

Gibbs, R. D. *Chemotaxonomy of Flowering Plants*. Montreal: McGill-Queens University Press, 1974.

Gifford, George E. "Botanic Remedies in Colonial Massachusetts, 1620–1820." *Medicine in Colonial Massachusetts, 1620–1820*. Ed. Philip Cash, Eric H. Christianson, and Worth J. Estes. Boston: Colonial Society of Massachusetts, 1980. 263–88.

Gilmore, Melvin R. *Uses of Plants by the Indians of the Missouri River Region*. U. S. Bureau of American Ethnology, 33d Annual Report, 1911–12. Washington: GPO, 1919.

Glass, James L. "Herbal Cures in the Fennell Diary." *North Carolina Folklore Journal* 31 (1983): 38–42.

Gordon, Lesley. *Green Magic: Flowers, Plants and Herbs in Lore and Legend*. New York: Viking, 1977.

Gosling, Nalda. *Herbs for Headaches and Migraine*. Wellingborough, Northamptonshire, England: Thorsons, 1978.

Griffin, LaDean. *No Side Effects: The Return to Herbal Medicine*. Provo, Utah: Bi-World, n.d.

Gunther, E. *Ethnobotany of Western Washington*. Seattle: University of Washington Press, 1977.

Guthrie, A. G. "Poisoning by Poke Root." *Journal of the American Medical Association* 9 (1887): 125.

Hatfield, Vivienne Gabrielle. "Herbs in Pregnancy, Childbirth, and Breastfeeding." *Plant-Lore Studies*. Ed. Roy Vickery. London: Folklore Society, 1984.

Heiser, Charles B., Jr. *Nightshades: The Paradoxical Plants*. San Francisco: Freeman, 1969.

Herbal Medicine Revisited. Special feature in *American Pharmacy*. Washington, D.C.: American Pharmaceutical Association, 1979.

Hilliard, Addie Suggs. "On Swallowing Punkin Seed." *Tennessee Folklore Society Bulletin* 40 (1974): 119–21.

Hirshhorn, H. H. "Botanical Remedies of South and Central America, and the Caribbean: An Archival Analysis." *Journal of Ethnopharmacology* 5 (1982): 163–80.

Hough, Walter. "Folk Medicine." *Journal of American Folklore* 15 (1902): 192.

Hufford, C. D., et al. "Two Antimicrobial Alkaloids from Heartwood of *Liriodendron tulipifera* L." *Journal of Pharmacological Science* 64.5 (1975): 789–92.

Hyams, C. W. "Medicinal Plants in North Carolina." *North Carolina Agricultural Experimental Station Bulletin* 150. Raleigh, 1898.

Inglis, Brian. *Natural Medicine*. London: Collins, 1979.

Jacobs, M. L., and H. M. Burlage. *Index of Plants of North Carolina with Reputed Medicinal Uses*. Chapel Hill, N.C.: Burlage, 1958.

Jolicoeur, Catherine. "Traditional Use of Herbs in Quebec." *The Potomac Herb Journal* 7 (1971): 3–5.

Jones, Olive R. "Essence of Peppermint: A History of the Medicine and Its Bottle." *Historical Archeologist* 15.2 (1981): 1–57.

Kirtikar, K. R., and B. D. Basu. *Indian Medicinal Plants*. 5 vols. Delhi: Jayyed, 1975.

Kordel, Lelord. *Natural Folk Remedies*. New York: Putnam, 1974.

Lawrence, G. H. M. *Taxonomy of Vascular Plants*. New York: Macmillan, 1951.

Li, C. P. *Chinese Herbal Medicine*. Bethesda, Md.: NIH, 1974.

Lloyd, J. U. "History of the Vegetable Drugs of the Pharmacopoeia of the United States." *Bulletin of the Lloyd Library* 18. Cincinnati, 1911.

Lornell, Kip. "'Sod' Rogers: Tipton County Herbalist." *Tennessee Folklore Society Bulletin* 48 (1982): 61–65.

Lucas, Richard. *Secrets of the Chinese Herbalists*. West Nyack, N.Y.: Parker, 1977.

Mairesse, Michelle. *Health Secrets of Medicinal Herbs*. New York: Arco, 1981.

Malone, E. T., Jr. "A Further Note on Herb Doctor Cicero West." *North Carolina Folklore Journal* 30 (1982): 52–53.

McClafferty, Brian. "On the Efficacy of Ginseng." *North Carolina Folklore* 20 (1972): 137–38.

Meyer, Clarence. *Vegetarian Medicines*. Glenwood, Ill.: Meyerbooks, 1981.

Miller, Amy Bess. *Shaker Herbs: A History and a Compendium*. New York: Crown, 1976.

Moerman, Daniel E. *Geraniums for the Iroquois: A Field Guide to American Indian Medicinal Plants*. Algonac, Mich.: Reference, 1982.

——. "Poisoned Apples and Honeysuckles: The Medicinal Plants of Native America." *Medical Anthropology Quarterly* 3.1 (1989): 52–61.

Morton, Julia F. *Major Medicinal Plants: Botany, Culture and Uses*. Springfield, Ill.: Thomas, 1977.

Mullins, Gladys. "Herbs of the Southern Highlands and Their Medicinal Uses." *Kentucky Folklore Record* 19 (1973): 36–41.

Myerhoff, Barbara G. *Peyote Hunt: The Sacred Journey of the Huichol Indians*. Ithaca, N.Y.: Cornell University Press, 1974.

Palmer, Edward. "Plants Used by the Indians of the United States." *American Naturalist* 12 (1878): 593–606.

Petkov, V. "Plants with Hypotensive, Antiatheromatous and Coronaroidilatating Action." *American Journal of Clinical Medicine* 7.3 (1979): 197–236.

Pope, Rita Tregellas. "Bean Lore." *Plant-Lore Studies*. Ed. Roy Vickery. London: Folklore Society, 1984. 139–47.

Robbins, Wilfred W., John P. Harrington, and Barbara Freire-Marreco. *Ethnobotany of the Tewa Indians*. Bureau of American Ethnology Bulletin 55. Washington: GPO, 1916.

Rogers, Dilwyn J. *Lakota Names and Traditional Uses of Native Plants by Sicangu (Brule) People in the Rosebud Area, South Dakota*. St. Francis, S.D.: Buechel Memorial Lakota Museum, 1980.

Romero, John Bruno. *The Botanical Lore of the California Indians with Side Lights on Historical Incidents in California* New York: Vantage, 1954.

Safford, W. E. "Narcotic Plants and Stimulants of the Ancient Americans." *Annual Report of the Smithsonian Institution 1916*. Washington, D.C.: GPO, 1917.

Schulles, Richard Evans. "Appeal of Peyote as a Medicine." *American Anthropologist* 40 (1938): 698–715.

Schuphan, W., and H. Weiller. "Investigations on the Antibacterial Effects of the Essential Oil of Carrots (Daucus Carota and Its Constituents)." *Biological Abstracts* 60 (1969): 1468–69.

Scully, Susan. *A Treasury of American Indian Herbs: Their Lore and Their Use for Food, Drugs, and Medicine*. New York: Crown, 1970.

Sherry, C. J., and J. A. Koontz. "Pharmacologic Studies of 'Catnip Tea': the Hot Water Extract of *Nepeta Cataria*." *Quarterly Journal of Crude Drug Research* 17 (1979): 68–72.

Sherry, C. J., T. W. Robinson, and K. Powell. "Catnip (*Nepeta Cataria*): an Evaluation of the Cold Water and Acetone-Pretreated Hot Water Extracts." *Quarterly Journal of Crude Drug Research* 19 (1981): 31–35.

Sheth, K., et al. "Phylochemical Investigation of the Leaves of *Chimaphila umbellata*" (abstract). *Lloydia* 29 (1966): 378.

Smith, Huron H. "Ethnobotany of the Forest Potawatomi Indians." *Bulletin of the Public Museum of Milwaukee* 7.1 (1933): 1–230.

——. "Ethnobotany of the Menomini Indians." *Bulletin of the Public Museum of Milwaukee* 4.1 (1923): 1–174.

——. "Ethnobotany of the Ojibwe Indians." *Bulletin of the Public Museum of Milwaukee* 4.3 (1932): 327–525.

Spoerke, David G., Jr. *Herbal Medications*. Santa Barbara, Calif.: Woodbridge, 1980.

Stevenson, Matilda C. "Ethnobotany of the Zuni Indians." *Thirtieth Annual Report, Bureau of American Ethnology 1908–1909*. Washington, D.C.: GPO, 1915.

Stewart, Omer C. "Peyotism and Mescaism." *Plains Anthropologist* 25 (1980): 297–309.

Stimson, Katherine. "Contributions Toward a Biography of the Medicinal Use of Plants by the Indians of the United States of America." MA Thesis, University of Pennsylvania, 1946.

Stoner, Michael. "Plantain: Its Uses as a Folk Remedy for Insect and Snake Bites." *Kentucky Folklore Record* 20 (1974): 96–98.

Strader, Clifton. "A Winston-Salem Folk Herbalist." *North Carolina Folklore Journal* 27 (1979): 20–25.

Sullivan, C. W. III. "Tobacco Medicine." *North Carolina Folklore Journal* 27 (1979): 26–31.

Tantaquidgeon, Gladys. "Notes on the Origin and Uses of Plants of Lake St. John Montagnais." *Journal of American Folklore* 45 (1932): 265–67.

Taylor, Dorothy Bright. "Indian Medicinal Herbs and the White Man's Medicine." *New York Folklore Quarterly* 23 (1967): 274–82.

Taylor, J. M. "Early Botanists and the Introduction of Drug Specifics." *Bulletin of the New York Academy of Medicine* 55 (1979): 684–99.

Tétényi, Péter. *Infraspecific Chemical Taxa of Medicinal Plants*. Budapest: Akadémiai Kiadó.

Thompson, Lawrence S. "Some Notes on the Folklore of Tobacco and Smoking." *Kentucky Folklore Record* 10 (1964): 43–46.

Tobe, John H. *The Golden Treasure of Natural Health Knowledge*. St. Catherines, Ontario: Provoker, 1973.

Trejo, Judy. "Medicinal and Edible Plants of the Paiute Indians." *Northwest Folklore* 4.1 (1985): 3–12.

Vartia, K. O. "Antibiotics in Lichens." *The Lichens*. Ed. Vernon Ahmadjian and Mason Hale. New York: Academic, 1973. 547–61.

Vestal, Paul K., Jr. "Herb Workers in Scotland and Robeson Counties." *North Carolina Folklore Journal* 21.4 (1973): 166–70.

Weiner, Michael. *Earth Medicine—Earth Foods: Plant Remedies, Drugs, and Natural Foods of the North American Indian*. New York: Collier, Macmillan, 1972.

Whiting, Alfred F. *Ethnobotany of the Hopi*. Flagstaff: Museum of Northern Arizona, 1966.

Willaman, J. J., and B. G. Schubert. "Alkaloid-Bearing Plants and Their Contained Alkaloids." *Agricultural Research Series. United States Department of Agriculture Technical Bulletin* 1234. Washington, D.C.: GPO, 1961.

Wilson, B. J., et al. "Perilla Ketone: A Potent Lung Toxin from the Mint Plant: *Perilla Frutescens* Britton." *Science* 197 (1977): 573–74.

Yoder, Don. "Herbs and Herb Lore: Folk-Cultural Questionnaire No. 25." *Pennsylvania Folklife* 21 (1971): inside front cover.

Zigmond, Maurice L. *Kawaiisu Ethnobotany*. Salt Lake City: University of Utah Press, 1981.

B. Magic, Witchcraft, Shamanism, and Charms

Anderson, John Q. "Magical Transference of Disease in Texas Folk Medicine." *Western Folklore* 27 (1968): 191–99.

Bandler, Richard, and John Grinder. *The Structure of Magic*. Palo Alto, Calif.: Science and Behavior Books, 1975.

Bayliss, Clara. "Witchcraft." *Journal of American Folklore* 21 (1908): 363.

Bean, Lowell John. "California Indian Shamanism and Folk Curing." *American Folk Medicine: A Symposium*. Ed. Wayland D. Hand. Berkeley: University of California Press, 1976. 108–25.

Bergman, Robert L. "A School for Medicine Men." *American Journal of Psychiatry* 130 (1973): 663–66.

Brown, Michael Fobes. "Shamanism and Its Discontents." *Medical Anthropology Quarterly* 2.2 (1988): 102–20.

Combs, Josiah. "Symbolic Magic in the Kentucky Mountains: Some Curious Folk Survivals." *Journal of American Folklore* 54 (1941): 328–30.

Creighton, Helen. *Bluenose Magic*. Toronto: Ryerson, 1968.

Crosby, John R. "Modern Witches of Pennsylvania." *Journal of American Folklore* 40 (1927): 304–9.

Cross, Tom Pete. "Witchcraft in North Carolina." *Studies in Philology* 16.3 (1919): 217–87.

Dixon, Roland. "Some Shamans of Northern California." *Journal of American Folklore* 17 (1904): 23–27.

Dow, James. *The Shaman's Touch: Otomi Indian Symbolic Healing*. Salt Lake City: University of Utah Press, 1986.

Eliade, Mircea. *Shamanisn: Archaic Techniques of Ecstasy*. Trans. W. R. Trask. Bollingen Series 76. New York: Pantheon, 1964.

Gandee, Lee R. *Strange Experience: The Secrets of a Hexenmeister*. Englewood Cliffs, N.J.: Prentice-Hall, 1971.

Hagar, Stansburg. "Micmac, Magic and Medicine." *Journal of American Folklore* 9 (1896): 170–77.

Hall, Manly P. "The American Indian Medicine Man." *The Story of Healing: The Divine Art*. New York: Citadel, 1958.

Hand, Wayland D. "Folk Medical Magic and Symbolism in the West." *Forms Upon the Frontier: Folklife and Folk Art in the United States*. Ed. Austin Fife, Alta Fife, and Henry Glassie. Monograph Series 16, no. 2. Logan: Utah State University Press, 1969. 103–18.

——. "Hangmen, the Gallows, and the Dead Man's Hand in American Folk Medicine." *Medieval Literature and Folklore Studies: Essays in Honor of Francis Lee Utley*. Ed. J. Mandel and B. A. Rosenberg. New Brunswick, N.J.: Rutgers University Press, 1970. 323–30.

——. "Magical Medicine: An Alternative to 'Alternative Medicine.'" *Western Folklore* 44 (1985): 240–51.

——. *Magical Medicine: The Folkloric Component of Medicine in the Folk Belief, Custom, and Ritual of the Peoples of Europe and America*. Berkeley: University of California Press, 1980.

——. "The Magical Transference of Disease." *North Carolina Folklore* 13 (1965): 83–111.

——. "Magical Treatment of Disease by Outlining the Ailing Part." *Bulletin of the New York Academy of Medicine* 48 (1972): 951–54.

——. "Measuring with String, Thread, and Fibre: A Practice in Folk Medical Magic." *Festschrift für Robert Wildhaber Zum 70*. Geburtstag am 3. Ed. Walter Escher, Theo Ganter, and Hans Trumpy. Basel: Verlag G. Krebs AG, 1973. 240–51.

——. "Onomastic Magic in the Health, Sickness, and Death of Man." *Names* 32.1 (1984): 1–13.

——. "Plugging, Nailing, Wedging and Kindred Folk Medical Practices." *Folklore and Society:*

Essays in Honor of Benjamin A. Botkin. Ed. B. Jackson. Hatboro, Penn.: Folklore Associates, 1966.

Harner, Michael J. *Hallucinogens and Shamanism*. New York: Oxford University Press, 1973.

Holland, William. "Mexican-American Medical Beliefs: Science or Magic." *Arizona Medicine* 20.5 (1963): 93.

Hufford, David J. "A New Approach to the 'Old Hag': The Nightmare Tradition Reexamined." *American Folk Medicine: A Symposium*. Ed. Wayland D. Hand. Berkeley: University of California Press, 1976. 73–87.

——. *The Terror That Comes in the Night: An Experience-Centered Study of Supernatural Assault Traditions*. Philadelphia, Penn.: University of Pennsylvania Press, 1982.

Kiev, Ari, ed. *Magic, Faith, and Healing*. New York: Free Press, 1964.

Kittredge, George Lyman. *Witchcraft in Old and New England*. 1929. New York: Atheneum, 1972.

Krech, Shepard, III. "'Throwing Bad Medicine': Sorcery, Disease and the Fur Trade Among the Kutchin and Other Northern Athapaskans." *Indians, Animals and the Fur Trade: A Critique of Keepers of the Game*. Ed. Shepard Krech, III. Athens: University of Georgia Press, 1981. 73–108.

LaFlesche, F. "The Omaha Buffalo Medicine Men." *Journal of American Folklore* 3 (1890): 215–21.

Long, Eleanor. "Aphrodisiacs, Charms, and Philtres." *Western Folklore* 32 (1973): 153–63.

MacColloch, J. A. "Shamanism." *James Hastings' Encyclopaedia of Religion and Ethics, 1908–1926*. N.p.

McTeer, J. E. *Fifty Years as a Low Country Witch-Doctor*. Columbia, S.C.: Bryan, 1976.

Middleton, John, ed. *Magic, Witchcraft, and Curing*. Garden City, N.Y.: Published for the American Museum of Natural History by the Natural History Press, 1967.

Miller, William Marion. "How to Become a Witch." *Journal of American Folklore* 57 (1944): 280.

Murphy, Jane M. "Psychotherapeutic Aspects of Shamanism on St. Lawrence Island, Alaska." *Magic, Faith, and Healing*. Ed. Ari Kiev. New York: Free Press, 1964. 53–83.

Myerhoff, Barbara G. "The Doctor as Culture Hero: The Shaman of Rincon." *Anthropological Quarterly* 39.2 (1966): 60–72.

——. "Shamanic Equilibrium: Balance and Mediation in Known and Unknown Worlds." *American Folk Medicine: A Symposium*. Ed. Wayland D. Hand. Berkeley: University of California Press, 1976. 99–109.

Noll, Richard. "Shamanism and Schizophrenia: A State-Specific Approach to the Schizophrenic Metaphor of Shamanic States." *American Ethnologist* 10 (1983): 443–59.

Opler, M. E. "Some Points of Comparison and Contrast Between the Treatment of Functional Disorders by Apache Shamans and Modern Psychiatric Practice." *American Journal of Psychiatry* 92 (1936): 1371–87.

Paredes, J. Anthony. "A Case Study of 'Normal' Windigo." *Anthropologica* 14 n.s. (1972): 97–116.

Pendleton, Louis. "Notes on Negro Folk-lore and Witchcraft in the South." *Journal of American Folklore* 3 (1890): 201–7.

Prince, Raymond. "Introduction to Shamans and Endorphins." *Ethos* 10.4 (1982): 299–302.

——. "Shamans and Endorphins: Hypotheses for a Synthesis." *Ethos* 10.4 (1982): 409–23.

Reichel-Dolmatoff, G. "Brain and Mind in Desana Shamanism." *Journal of Latin American Lore* 7.1 (1981): 73–98.

Rickels, Patricia. "Some Accounts of Witch Riding." *Lousiana Folklore Miscellany* 2.1 (1961): 1–17.

Robbins, Rossell. *The Encyclopedia of Witchcraft and Demonology*. London: Hamlin, 1959.

Santino, Jack, ed. "Healing, Magic and Religion." *Western Folklore* (Special Issue) 44.3 (1985): 153–253.

Snow, Loudell F. "Mail-Order Magic: The Commercial Exploitation of Folk Belief." *Journal of the Folklore Institute* 16 (1979): 44–74.

——. "Voodoo Illness in the Black Population." *Culture, Curers, and Contagion*. Ed. Norman Klein. Novato, Calif.: Chandler and Sharp, 1979. 179–84.

Torrey, E. Fuller. *The Mind Game: Witchdoctors and Psychiatrists*. New York: Emerson, 1972.

Townsend, Barbara Ann, and Donald Allport Bird. "The Miracle of String Measurement." *Indiana Folklore* 3 (1970): 147–62.

Vickers, Ovid. "Choctaw Medicine Men: The Practice Continues." *Mississippi Folklore Register* 15 (1981): 51–56.

Wilson, Gordon. "Talismans and Magic in Folk Remedies in the Mammoth Cave Region." *Southern Folklore Quarterly* 30 (1966): 192–201.

Winkelman, Michael J. "Shamans and Other 'Magico-Religious' Healers: A Cross-Cultural Study of Their Origins, Nature, and Social Transformations." *Ethos* 18 (1990): 305–52.

C. Rootwork, Voodoo, Conjuring, and Spiritualism

Bacon, A. M. "Conjuring and Conjure-Doctors in the Southern United States." *Journal of American Folklore* 9 (1896): 143–47, 224–26.

Beynon, E. D. "The Voodoo Cult Among Negro Migrants in Detroit." *American Journal of Sociology* 43 (1938): 894–907.

Brown, Hugh S. "Voodooism in Northwest Louisiana." *Lousiana Folklore Miscellany* 2.2 (1965): 86.

Byers, James F. "Voodoo: Tropical Pharmacology or Psychosomatic Psychology?" *New York Folklore Quarterly* 26 (1970): 305–12.

Calin, Stewart. "Negro Sorcery in the United States." *Journal of American Folklore* 3 (1890): 281–87.

de Albuquerque, Klaus. "Folk Medicine in the South Carolina Sea Islands." *Proceedings of a Symposium on Culture and Health: Implications for Health Policy in Rural South Carolina*. Ed. Melba S. Varner. Charleston, S.C.: College of Charleston Center for Metropolitan Affairs and Public Policy, 1979. 33–79.

Hark, Ann. *Hex Marks the Spot in the Pennsylvania Dutch Country*. Philadelphia: Lippincott, 1938.

Harwood, Alan. *RX: Spiritist as Needed: A Study of a Puerto Rican Community Mental Health Resource*. New York: Wiley, 1977.

Herron, Leonora, and Alice M. Bacon. "Conjuring and Conjure Doctors." *Mother Wit from the Laughing Barrel: Readings in the Interpretation of Afro-American Folklore*. Ed. Alan Dundes. Englewood Cliffs, N.J.: Prentice-Hall, 1973. 359–68.

Heyer, Kathryn W. "Some Psychological Implications of Changing Medical Practice on the Sea Islands." *Proceedings of a Symposium on Culture and Health: Implications for Health Policy in Rural South Carolina*. Ed. Melba S. Varner. Charleston, S.C.: College of Charleston Center for Metropolitan Affairs and Public Policy, 1979.

Hurston, Zora Neale. "Hoodoo in America." *Journal of American Folklore* 44 (1931): 317–417.

Johnson, F. Roy. *The Fabled Doctor Jim Jordan: A Story of Conjure*. Murfreesboro, N.C.: Johnson, 1963.

Kilpatrick, Jack Frederick, and Anna Kilpatrick. "A Cherokee Conjuration to Cure a Horse." *Southern Folklore Quarterly* 28 (1964): 216–18.

Kuna, Ralph R. "Hoodoo: The Indigenous Medicine and Psychiatry of the Black American." *Ethnomedicine* 3 (1974): 273–94.

McLean, Patricia S. "Conjure Doctors in Eastern North Carolina." *North Carolina Folklore* 20 (1972): 21–29.

Mellinger, Marie B. "The Spirit Is Strong in the Root." *Appalachian Journal* 4 (1977): 242–54.

Rocereto, LaVerne R. "Rootwork and the Root Doctor." *Nursing Forum* 12 (1973): 414–26.

Snow, Loudell F. "Con Men and Conjure Men: A Ghetto Image." *Literature and Medicine* 2 (1983): 45–78.

——. "'I Was Born Just Exactly with the Gift': An Interview with a Voodoo Practitioner." *Journal of American Folklore* 86 (1973): 272–81.

Steiner, Roland. "Observations on the Practice of Conjuring in Georgia." *Journal of American Folklore* 14 (1901): 173–80.

Stitt, V. J. "Rootdoctors as Providers of Primary Care." *Journal of the National Medical Association* 75 (1983): 719–21.

Straight, William W. "Throw Downs, Fixin, Rooting and Hexing." *Journal of the Florida Medical Association* 70 (1983): 635–41.

Walker, Willard. "Cherokee Curing and Conjuring, Identity, and the Southeastern Co-Tradition." *Persistent Peoples: Cultural Enclaves in Perspective*. Ed. George Pierre Castile and Gilbert Kushner. Tucson: University of Arizona Press, 1981. 86–105.

Webb, Bernie Larson. "A Study of Voodoo Mail-Order Advertising in Louisiana." *Louisiana Review* 2 (1973): 68.

Webb, Julie Yvonne. "Louisiana Voodoo and Superstitions Related to Health." *HSMHA Health Reports* 86 (1971): 291–301.

Wintrob, Ronald M., and R. Fox. "Rootwork Beliefs and Psychological Disorders Among Blacks in a Northern United States City." *Proceedings of the Fifth World Congress of Psychology*. Mexico City, 1971.

D. Religious and Faith Healing

Amundsen, Darrel W., and Gary B. Ferngren. "Medicine and Religion: Early Christianity Through the Middle Ages." *Health/Medicine and the Faith Traditions: An Inquiry into Religion and Medicine*. Ed. Martin E. Marty and Kenneth Vaux. Philadelphia: Fortress, 1982. 93–132.

Anonymous. "Home Remedies." *The Foxfire Book*. Ed. Eliot Wigginton. Garden City, N.Y.: Doubleday, 1972. 230–48.

Baer, Hans A. "Prophets and Advisors in Black Spiritual Churches: Therapy, Pallative, or Opiate?" *Culture, Medicine, and Psychiatry* 5 (1981): 145–70.

Bourguignon, Erica. "The Effectiveness of Religious Healing Movements: A Review of the Literature." *Transcultural Psychiatric Research Review* 13 (1976): 5–21.

Calestro, Kenneth. "Psychotherapy, Faith Healing, and Suggestion." *International Journal of Psychiatry* 10.2 (1972): 83–113.

Clements, William M. "Faith Healing Narratives from Northeast Arkansas." *Indiana Folklore* 9 (1976): 15–39.

——. "Ritual Expectation in Pentecostal Healing Experience." *Western Folklore* 40 (1981): 139–48.

Csordas, Thomas J. "Elements of Charismatic Persuasion and Healing." *Medical Anthropology Quarterly* 2 (1988): 121–42.

——. "The Rhetoric of Transformation in Ritual Healing." *Culture, Medicine, and Psychiatry* 7 (1983): 333–75.

Delgado, Melvin. "Puerto Rican Spiritualism and the Social Work Profession." *Social Case Work* (October 1977): 451–58.

Faith Healing. A special issue of the *British Medical Journal* (1910): 1453–1502.

"Faith Healing." *Foxfire 1* (1968): 15–24, 61–70.

Favazza, Armando R. "Modern Christian Healing of Mental Illness." *American Journal of Psychiatry* 139 (1982): 728–35.

Fishman, Robert Gary. "Spiritualism in Western New York: A Study in Ritual Healing." *Medical Anthropology* 3 (1979): 1–22.

Frazier, Claude A., ed. *Faith Healing: Finger of God? Or Scientific Curiosity?* New York: Nelson, 1973.

Gopalan, G. V., coll., and Bruce E. Nickerson, ed. "Faith Healing in Indiana and Illinois." *Indiana Folklore* 6 (1973): 33–99.

Harrell, David Erwin, Jr. *All Things Are Possible: The Healing and Charismatic Revivals in Modern America*. Bloomington: Indiana University Press, 1975.

Hufford, David J. "Christian Religious Healing." *Journal of Operational Psychiatry* 8.2 (1977): 22–27.

——. "Sainte Anne de Beaupré: Roman Catholic Pilgrimage and Healing." *Western Folklore* 44 (1985): 194–207.

Jackson, Edgar N. *The Role of Faith in the Process of Healing*. Minneapolis: Winston, 1981.

John, De Witt. *The Christian Science Way of Life*. Englewood Cliffs, N.J.: Prentice-Hall, 1963.

Johnson, Greg. "A Classification of Faith Healing Practices." *New York Folklore* 1 (1975): 91–96.

Jones, Michael Owen. *Why Faith Healing?* National Museum of Man, National Museums of Canada, Canadian Center for Folk Culture Studies, Mercury Series, no. 3. Ottawa, 1972.

Kelsey, Morton. *Healing and Christianity: In Ancient Thought and Modern Times*. New York: Harper and Row, 1973.

Kerewsky-Halpern, Barbara. "Talk, Touch, and Trust in Rural Healing." *Papers for the Fifth Congress of Southeast European Studies*. Belgrade, September, 1984. Ed. Kot K. Shangriladze and Erica W. Townsend. Columbus, Ohio: Slavica for U.S. National Committee of AIESEE, 1984.

Maki, Lillian. *Mother, God, and Mental Health*. Portland: Metropolitan, 1980.

Marty, Martin E., and Kenneth L. Vaux, eds. *Health/Medicine and the Faith Traditions: An Inquiry into Religion and Medicine*. Philadelphia: Fortress, 1982.

Miller, Heather Ross. "The Palmer Christian." *North Carolina Folklore Journal* 24 (1976): 75–81.

Miller, Jim Wayne. "More About Faith Healers." *North Carolina Folklore* 17 (1969): 97–99.

Pattison, E. Mansell, Nikolajs A. Lapins, and Hans A. Doerr. "Faith Healing: A Study of Personality and Function." *Journal of Nervous and Mental Disease* 157 (1973): 397–409.

Raichelson, Richard M. "Belief and Effectivity: Folk Medicine in Tennessee." *Tennessee Folklore Society Bulletin* 49 (1983): 103–19.

Schoepflin, Rennie B. "Christian Science Healing in America." *Other Healers: Unorthodox Medicine in America*. Ed. Norman Genitz. Baltimore: Johns Hopkins University Press, 1988. 192–214.

Simson, Eve. *The Faith Healer: Deliverance Evangelism in North America*. New York: Pyramid, 1977.

Singer, Philip, ed. *Traditional Healing: New Science or New Colonialism*. Buffalo, N.Y.: Conch, 1977.

Snow, Loudell F. "The Religious Component in Southern Folk Medicine." *Traditional Healing: New Science or New Colonialism*. Ed. Philip Singer. Buffalo, N.Y.: Conch, 1977. 26–51.

Teske, Robert T. "Votive Offerings and the Belief System of Greek-Philadelphians." *Western Folklore* 44 (1985): 208–24.

Tillich, Paul. "The Relation of Religion and Healing." *The Review of Religion* 10 (1946): 348–84.

Wigginton, Eliot. "Two Faith Healers Tell Exactly How It's Done." *North Carolina Folklore Journal* 16 (1968): 163–65.

E. Psychosomatic Conditions and Hypnosis

Adler, Herbert M., and Van Buren O. Hammett. "The Doctor-Patient Relationship Revisited: An Analysis of the Placebo Effect. *Annals of Internal Medicine* 78 (1973): 595–98.

Beecher, H. K. "Increased Stress and Effectiveness of Placebos and 'Active' Drugs." *Science* 132 (1960): 91–92.

——. "The Powerful Placebo." *Journal of the American Medical Association* 159 (1955): 1602–6.

——. "Surgery as Placebo." *Journal of the American Medical Association* 176 (1961): 1102–7.

Benson, H., and M. D. Epstein. "The Placebo Effect: A Neglected Asset in the Care of Patients." *Journal of the American Medical Association* 232 (1975): 1275–77.

Brody, H. *Placebos and the Philosophy of Medicine: Clinical, Conceptual, and Ethical Issues*. Chicago: University of Chicago Press, 1980.

Byerly, Henry. "Explaining and Exploiting Placebo Effects." *Perspectives in Biology and Medicine* 19 (1976): 423–36.

Carter, D. B., and D. Allen. "Evaluation of the Placebo Effect in Optometry." *American Journal of Optometry* 50 (1973): 99–103.

Clark, W. G., and J. del Guidice, eds. *Principles of Psychopharmacology*. New York: Academic, 1970.

Claus, Edward P. *Gathercoal and Wirth Pharmacognosy*. 3d ed. revised. Philadelphia: Lea and Febiger, 1956.

Lipowski, Z. J., Don Lipsett, and Peter Whybrow, eds. *Psychosomatic Medicine: Current Trends and Clinical Applications*. New York: Oxford University Press, 1977.

Moerman, Daniel E. "Physiology and Symbols: The Anthropological Implications of the Placebo Effect." *The Anthropology of Medicine: From Culture to Method*. Ed. L. Romanucci-Ross, D. Moerman, and L. Tancredi. New York: Praeger, 1983. 156–67.

Ness, Robert C., and Ronald M. Wintrob. "Folk Healing: A Description and Synthesis." *American Journal of Psychiatry* 138 (1981): 1477–81.

Price, Douglas B. "Miraculous Restoration of Lost Body Parts: Relationship to the Phantom Limb Phenomenon and the Limb-Burial Superstitions and Practices." *American Folk Medicine: A Symposium*. Ed. Wayland D. Hand. Berkeley: University of California Press, 1976. 49–73.

Schwab, John H., Eileen Fennell, and George Warheit. "The Epidemiology of Psychosomatic Disorders." *Psychosomatics* 15 (1974): 88–93.

Snell, John E. "Hypnosis in the Treatment of the Hexed Patient." *Journal of Psychiatry* 124.3 (1967): 311–16.

Virtanen, Leea. "Psychic Disturbances: Views on Etiology and Care." *Folk Medicine and Health Culture: Role of Folk Medicine in Modern Health Care*. Ed. Tuula Vaskilampi and Carol MacCormack. Kuopio, Finland: University of Kuopio Press, 1982. 28–39.

F. Ethnopsychiatry, Psychotherapy, Symbolic Healing, and Nervios

Bateson, Gregory. *Steps to an Ecology of Mind*. North Vale, N.J.: Aronson, 1987.

Benor, Daniel J. "Psychic Healing." *Alternative Medicines: Popular and Policy Perspectives*. Ed. J. Warren Salmon. New York: Tavistock, 1984. 165–90.

Berne, Eric. "The Mythology of Dark and Fair: Psychiatric Use of Folklore." *Journal of American Folklore* 72 (1959): 1–13.

Bohart, Arthur C. "Toward a Cognitive Theory of Catharsis." *Psychotherapy: Theory, Research, and Practice* 17.2 (1980): 192–201.

Devereux, George. *Mohave Ethnopsychiatry: The Psychic Disturbances of an Indian Tribe*. Washington, D.C.: Smithsonian, 1969.

Douglas, Mary. *Purity and Danger: An Analysis of Concepts of Pollution and Taboo*. Harmondsworth, England: Penguin, 1970.

Dow, James. "Universal Aspects of Symbolic Healing: A Theoretical Synthesis." *American Anthropologist* 88 (1986): 56–69.

Elliott, Robert. "A Discovery-Oriented Approach to Significant Change Events in Psychotherapy: Interpersonal Process Recall and Comprehensive Process Analysis." *Patterns of Change*. Ed. Laura Rice and Leslie Greenberg. New York: Guilford, 1984. 249–86.

Epstein, Gerald N. "The Experience of Waking Dream in Psychotherapy." *Healing: Implications for Psychotherapy*. Ed. James Fosshage and Paul Olsen. New York: Human Sciences, 1978. 137–84.

Fosshage, James, and Paul Olsen, eds. *Healing: Implications for Psychotherapy*. New York: Human Sciences, 1978.

Foster, George M. "The Anatomy of Envy: A Study in Symbolic Behavior." *Current Anthropology* 13 (1972): 165–202.

Foulks, Edward, and Frances Schwartz. "Self and Object: Psychoanalytical Perspectives in Cross-Cultural Fieldwork and Interpretation: A Review Essay." *Ethos* 10.3 (1982): 254–78.

Frank, Jerome D. *Persuasion and Healing: A Comparative Study of Psychotherapy*. Baltimore: Johns Hopkins University Press, 1961. New York: Schocken, 1967.

——. "Physiotherapy of Bodily Diseases: An Overview." *Psychotherapy and Psychosomatics* 26 (1975): 192–202.

——. "Therapeutic Components of Psychotherapy." *Journal of Nervous and Mental Disease* 159 (1974): 325–42.

Garrison, Vivian. "Doctor, *Espiritista*, or Psychiatrist? Health-Seeking Behavior in a Puerto Rican Neighborhood of New York City." *Medical Anthropology* 1.2 (1977): 65–191.

——. "Folk Healing Systems as Elements in the Community Support Systems of Psychiatric Patients." *Therapeutic Interventions: Healing Strategies for Human Systems*. Ed. Uri Rueveni, Ross V. Speck, and Joan Speck. New York: Human Sciences, 1982. 58–95.

Harwood, Alan. "Puerto Rican Spiritism: An Institution with Preventive and Therapeutic Functions in Community Psychiatry." *Culture, Medicine, and Psychiatry* 1 (1977): 135–53.

Jenkins, J. H. "Ethnopsychiatric Interpretations of Schizophrenic Illness: The Problem of Nervios Within the Mexican-American Family." *Culture, Medicine, and Psychiatry* 12 (1988): 301–29.

Kennedy, John G. "Ethnopsychiatry, or Transcultural Psychiatry." *Teaching Medical Anthropology: Model Courses for Graduate and Undergraduate Instruction*. Ed. Harry F. Todd, Jr., and Julio L. Ruffini. Washington, D.C.: Society for Medical Anthropology, 1979. 75–94.

Kiev, Ari. *Curanderismo: Mexican-American Folk Psychiatry*. 1968. New York: Free Press, 1972.

——. "The Psychotherapeutic Aspects of Primitive Medicine." *Human Organization* 21 (1962): 25–29.

——. "The Study of Folk Psychiatry." *Magic, Faith, and Healing*. Ed. Ari Kiev. New York: Free Press, 1964.

Kleinman, Arthur. "Medicine's Symbolic Reality." *Inquiry* 16 (1973): 206–13.

Krippner, Stanley. "Psychic Healing." *Health for the Whole Person: The Complete Guide to Holistic Medicine*. Ed. Arthur C. Hastings, James Fadiman, and James S. Gordon. Boulder, Colo.: Westview, 1980. 169–71.

La Barre, Weston. "Confession as Cathartic Therapy in American Indian Tribes." *Magic, Faith, and Healing*. Ed. Ari Kiev. New York: Free Press, 1964.

Labov, William, and David Fanshel. *Therapeutic Discourse: Psychotherapy as Conversation*. New York: Academic, 1977.

Moerman, Daniel E. "Anthropology of Symbolic Healing." *Current Anthropology* 20 (1979): 59–80.

Obrist, Paul A., et al. *Cardiovascular Psychophysiology: Current Issues in Response Mechanisms, Biofeedback, and Methodology*. New York: Plenum, 1981.

Pattison, E. Mansell. "Exorcism and Psychotherapy: A Case of Collaboration." *Religious Systems and Psychotherapy*. Ed. Richard H. Cox. Springfield, Ill.: Thomas, 1973.

Prince, Raymond. "Psychotherapy as the Manipulation of Endogenous Healing Mechanisms: A Transcultural Survey." *Transcultural Psychiatric Research Review* 13 (1976): 115–33.

——. "Variations in Psychotherapeutic Procedures." *Handbook of Cross-Cultural Psychology*. Ed. Harry C. Triandis and Juris G. Draguns. Vol. 6. Boston: Allyn, 1980. 291–349.

White, Geoffrey M. "The Ethnographic Study of Cultural Knowledge of 'Mental Disorder.'" *Cultural Conceptions of Mental Health and Therapy*. Ed. Anthony Marsella and Geoffrey M. White. Boston: Reidel, 1982. 69–95.

Wiedorn, William S., Jr. "Psychotherapeutic-like Technique in Folk Medicine." *Louisiana Folklore Miscellany* 1.3 (1958): 11–20.

G. Menstruation, Pregnancy, Childbirth and Children, Midwifery

Bass, William W. "Birthmarks Among the Folk." *Tennessee Folklore Society Bulletin* 25 (1959): 1–6.

Beckwith, Martha Warren. "Function and Meaning of the Kumulipo Birth Chant in Ancient Hawaii." *Journal of American Folklore* 62 (1949): 290–93.

Bromberg, Joann. "Having a Baby: A Story Essay." *Childbirth: Alternatives to Medical Control*. Ed. Shelly Romalis. Austin: University of Texas Press, 1981. 33–62.

Brown, Judith K. "A Cross-Cultural Exploration of the End of the Child-Bearing Years." *Changing Perspectives on Menopause*. Ed. Ann M. Voda, Myra Dinnerstein, and Sheryl R. O'Donnell. Austin: University of Texas Press, 1982. 51–59.

Buckley, Thomas. "Menstruation and the Power of Yurok Women: Methods in Cultural Reconstruction." *American Ethnologist* 9.1 (1982): 47–60.

Buckley, Thomas, and Alma Gottlieb, eds. *Blood Magic: The Anthropology of Menstruation*. Berkeley: University of California Press, 1988.

Campbell, Marie. *Folks Do Get Born*. New York: Garland, 1984.

Cochran, Robert, and Martha Cochran. "Some Menstrual Folklore of Mississippi (Interviews Done in Marion County)." *Mississippi Folklore Register* 4 (1970): 108–13.

Dougherty, Molly C. "Southern Midwifery and Organized Health Care: Systems in Conflict." *Medical Anthropology* 6 (1982): 113–26.

Eccles, Audrey. *Obstetrics and Gynaecology in Tudor and Stuart England*. Kent, Ohio: Kent State University Press, 1982.

Ehrenreick, Barbara, and Deirdre English. *Complaints and Disorders: The Sexual Politics of Sickness*. New York: Feminist Press, 1973.

Farr, T. J. "Tennessee Folk Beliefs Concerning Children." *Journal of American Folklore* 52 (1939): 112–16.

Fife, Austin E. "Birthmarks and Psychic Imprinting of Babies in Utah Folk Medicine." *American Folk Medicine: A Symposium*. Ed. Wayland D. Hand. Berkeley: University of California Press, 1976. 273–84.

Fish, Lydia. "The Old Wife in the Dormitory—Sexual Folklore and Magical Practices from State University College." *New York Folklore Quarterly* 28 (1972): 30–36.

Forbes, Thomas R. *The Midwife and the Witch*. New Haven, Conn.: Yale University Press, 1966.

Frankel, Barbara. *Childbirth in the Ghetto: Folk Beliefs of Negro Women in a North Philadelphia Hospital Ward*. San Francisco: R and E Research, 1977.

Freedman, Alex S. "The Passing of the Arkansas Granny Midwife." *Kentucky Folklore Record* 20 (1974): 101–4.

Friedman, Albert B. "Grounding a Superstition: Lactation as Contraceptive." *Journal of American Folklore* 95 (1982): 200–208.

Hanawalt, Barbara A. "Conception Through Infancy in Medieval English Historical and Folklore Sources." *Folklore Forum* 13 (1980): 127–57.

Hand, Wayland D., et al. "Birth, Infancy, Childhood." *Popular Beliefs and Superstitions: A Compendium of American Folklore*. Boston: Hall, 1981.

Hartland, E. Sidney. "Cleft Ashes for Infantile Hernia." *Folk-lore* 7 (1896): 303–6.

Johnson, Shirley M., and Loudell F. Snow. "Assessment of Reproductive Knowledge in an Inner-City Clinic." *Social Science and Medicine* 16 (1982): 1657–62.

Johnstone, H. B. "Diseases of Children." *Journal of American Folklore* 16 (1903): 189–90.

Jordan, Brigitte. "Studying Childbirth: The Experience and Methods of a Woman Anthropologist." *Childbirth: Alternatives to Medical Control*. Ed. Shelley Romalis. Austin: University of Texas Press, 1981. 181–216.

Kamsler, Harold. "Hebrew Menstrual Taboos." *Journal of American Folklore* 51 (1938): 76–82.

Kobrin, Frances E. "The American Midwife Controversy: A Crisis of Professionalization." *Bulletin of the History of Medicine* 40.4 (1966): 350–63.

McClain, Carol. "Traditional Midwives and Family Planning: An Assessment of Programs and Suggestions for the Future." *Medical Anthropology* 5.1 (1981): 107–36.

McIntosh, Karyl. "Folk Obstetrics, Gynecology, and Pediatrics in Utica, New York." *New York Folklore* 4 (1978): 49–59.

Manderson, Lenore. "Roasting, Smoking and Dieting in Response to Birth: Malay Confinement in Cross-Cultural Perspective." *Social Science and Medicine* 15B (1981): 509–20.

Mathews, Holly F. "Killing the Medical Self-Help Tradition among African-Americans: The Case of Lay Midwifery in North Carolina, 1912–1983." *African-Americans in the South: Issues of Race, Class, and Gender*. Ed. Hans Baer and Yvonne Jones. Athens, Ga.: University of Georgia Press, 1992.

Meigs, Joseph A. "Choosing Your Baby's Sex—Now and in the Sixteenth Century." *Tennessee Folklore Society Bulletin* 48 (1982): 111–16.

Mongeau, Beatrice, et al. "The 'Granny' Midwife: Changing Roles and Functions of a Folk Practitioner." *American Journal of Sociology* 66 (1961): 497–501.

Murphy, Charles H. "A Collection of Birth Marking Beliefs from Eastern Kentucky." *Kentucky Folklore Record* 10 (1964): 36–38.

Newman, Lucile F. "Folklore of Pregnancy: Wives' Tales in Contra Costa County, California." *Western Folklore* 28 (1969): 112–35.

Newman, Lucile F., ed. "Midwives and Modernization." *Medical Anthropology* 5.1 (1981): 1–12.

Radbill, Samuel X. "Child Hygiene Among the American Indians: A Chapter in Early American Pediatrics." *Texas Reports on Biology and Medicine* 3 (1945): 419–512.

——. "The Folklore of Teething." *Keystone Folklore Quarterly* 9 (1964): 123–43.

——. "The Role of Animals in Infant Feeding." *American Folk Medicine: A Symposium.* Ed. Wayland D. Hand. Berkeley: University of California Press, 1976. 21–30.

——. "Whooping Cough in Fact and Fancy." *Bulletin of the History of Medicine* 13 (1943): 33–53.

Rolleston, J. D. "The Folklore of Children's Diseases." *Folk-Lore* 54 (1943): 287–307.

Romalis, Coleman. "Taking Care of the Little Woman: Father-Physician Relations During Pregnancy and Childbirth." *Childbirth: Alternatives to Medical Control.* Ed. Shelley Romalis. Austin: University of Texas Press, 1981. 92–121.

Romalis, Shelley. "Natural Childbirth and the Reluctant Physician." *Childbirth: Alternatives to Medical Control.* Ed. Shelley Romalis. Austin: University of Texas Press, 1981. 63–91.

——. "An Overview." *Childbirth: Alternatives to Medical Control.* Ed. Shelley Romalis. Austin: University of Texas Press, 1981. 3–32.

Romalis, Shelley, ed. *Childbirth: Alternatives to Medical Control.* Austin: University of Texas Press, 1981.

Sample, L. L., and Albert Mohr. "Wishram Birth and Obstetrics." *Ethnology* 19 (1980): 427–45.

Smith, Elmer L., and John Stewart. "The Mill as a Preventive and Cure of Whooping Cough." *Journal of American Folklore* 77 (1964): 76–77.

Snow, Loudell F., and Shirley M. Johnson. "Folklore, Food, Female Reproductive Cycle." *Ecology of Food and Nutrition* 7 (1978): 41–49.

——. "Modern Day Menstrual Folklore: Some Clinical Implications. *Journal of the American Medical Association* 237 (1977): 2736–39.

Spears, James E. "Negro Folk Maternal-Natal Care, Practices, and Remedies: A Glossary." *Mississippi Folklore Register* 5 (1971): 19–22.

——. "Some Negro Pregnancy Euphemisms and Birth Superstitions." *Mississippi Folklore Register* 4 (1970): 24–27.

Velimirovic, Helga, and Boris Velimirovic. "The Role of Traditional Birth Attendants in Health Services." *Medical Anthropology* 5.1 (1981): 89–105.

Voda, Ann M., Myra Dinnerstein, and Sheryl R. O'Donnel, eds. *Changing Perspectives on Menopause.* Austin: University of Texas Press, 1982.

Wood, Irene Hansel. "The Folk Medicine of Childbirth in the English and Scottish Ballads." *Tennessee Folklore Society Bulletin* 47 (1981): 25–29.

Wright, Ann L. "Variation in Navajo Menopause: Toward an Explanation." *Changing Perspectives on Menopause.* Ed. Ann M. Voda, Myra Dinnerstein, and Sheryl R. O'Donnell. Austin: University of Texas Press, 1982. 84–99.

H. Home Remedy, Popular Belief/Superstition, Madstones and Waters

Anderson, John Q. "Popular Beliefs in Texas, Louisiana, and Arkansas." *Southern Folklore Quarterly* 32 (1968): 304–19.

——. "Special Powers in Folk Cures and Remedies." *Tire Shrinker to Dragster*. Ed. Wilson M. Hudson. Austin, Tex.: Encino, 1968. 163–74.

Bauer, William W. *Potions, Remedies, and Old Wives Tales*. Garden City, N.Y.: Doubleday, 1969.

Booker, Elsie H., and Curtis Booker. "Patent Medicines Before the Wiley Act of 1906." *North Carolina Folklore* 18 (1970): 130–42.

Bourke, John G. "Popular Medicine, Customs, and Superstitions of the Rio Grande." *Journal of American Folklore* 7 (1894): 119–46.

Brewster, Paul G. "Folk Cures and Preventives from Southern Indiana." *Southern Folklore Quarterly* 3 (1939): 33–43.

Broadrick, Estelle D. "Old Folk Sayings and Home-Cures." *Tennessee Folklore Society Bulletin* 44 (1978): 35–36.

Brown, Roy M. "Treatment of Snake-Bite in Chapel Hill." *North Carolina Folklore* 4 (1956): 1.

Browne, Ray B. *Popular Beliefs and Practices from Alabama*. Folklore Studies 9. Berkeley: University of California Press, 1958.

Byington, Robert H. "Popular Beliefs and Superstitions from Pennsylvania." *Keystone Folklore Quarterly* 9.1 (1964): 3–12.

Cansler, Loman D. "Madstones and Hydrophobia." *Western Folklore* 23 (1964): 95–105.

Caroland, Emma Jean. "Popular Beliefs and Superstitions Known to Students of Clarksville High School." *Tennessee Folklore Society Bulletin* 28 (1962): 37–47.

Carter, Mary. "Home Remedies for Lung Congestion." *Journal of the Ohio Folklore Society* December 1972: 50.

Carter, Roland D. "Mountain Superstitions." *Tennessee Folklore Society Bulletin* 10.1 (1944): 1–6.

Case, Richard G. "'A True and Genuine Madstone.'" *New York Folklore Quarterly* 26 (1970): 297–304.

Clark, J. D. "Madstones in North Carolina." *North Carolina Folklore Journal* 24 (1976): 3–40.

——. "More Madstones in North Carolina." *North Carolina Folklore Journal* 25 (1977): 33–35.

——. "North Carolina Madstones: A Second and Final Supplement. *North Carolina Folklore Journal* 29 (1981): 106–7.

——. "North Carolina Superstitions." *North Carolina Folklore* 14 (1966): 3–40.

——. "Passing Through: A Folk Remedy." *North Carolina Folklore Journal* 23 (1975): 11–15.

——. "Quilling or Snuffing." *North Carolina Folklore* 19 (1971): 105–6.

Collins, Yandell, Jr. "Superstition and Belief Tales from Louisville." *Kentucky Folklore Record* 4 (1958): 71–78.

Cook, Janice. "Folk Remedies as Practiced in Central Mississippi." *Mississippi Folklore Register* 9 (1975): 197–200.

Cooke, Mrs. R. C., Mrs. E. D. Hamner, and Ben Gray Lumpkin. "Remedies." *Tennessee Folklore Society Bulletin* 42 (1976): 65–69.

Craft, Betty. "Superstitions from Frenchburg, Kentucky." *Kentucky Folklore Record* 10 (1964): 12–17.

de Lys, Claudia. *A Treasury of American Superstitions*. New York: Philosophical Library, 1949.

Dobie, J. F. "Madstones and Hydrophobia Skunks." *Madstones and Twisters*. Ed. M. C. Boatright, W. M. Hudson, and Allen Maxwell. Dallas: Southern Methodist University Press, 1958. 3–17.

Doering, J. Frederick. "Folk Remedies for Diverse Allergies." *Journal of American Folklore* 57 (1944): 140–41.

Driver, Harold E. "A Method of Investigating Individual Differences in Folkloristic Beliefs and Practices." *Midwest Folklore* 1 (1951): 99–105.

Dulles, C. W. "The Mad Stone." *Journal of the American Medical Association* 34 (1900): 1208–9.

Ericson, Eston Everett. "Madstones in North Carolina." *Folklore* (London) 49 (1938): 165–66.

Farr, T. J. "Riddles and Superstitions of Middle Tennessee." *Journal of American Folklore* 48 (1935): 318–36.

Fish, Lydia. "The Folklorist and Belief." *New York Folklore* (Special Issue) 8.3–4 (1982): 1–107.

Fogel, E. M. *Beliefs and Superstitions of the Pennsylvania Germans*. Philadelphia: Americana Germanica, 1915.

Forbes, Thomas R. "Lapis Bufonis: The Growth and Decline of a Medical Superstition." *Yale Journal of Biology and Medicine* 45 (1972): 139–49.

——. "The Madstone." *American Folk Medicine: A Symposium*. Ed. Wayland D. Hand. Berkeley: University of California Press, 1976. 11–20.

Graubard, Mark. "Some Contemporary Observations on Ancient Superstitions." *Journal of American Folklore* 59 (1946): 124–33.

Griffin, Hazel. "Folk Remedies of the Roanoke-Chowan Section." *North Carolina Folklore* 6 (1958): 30–31.

Guinn, Leon. "Home Remedies from Curry County." *Texas Folklore Society Publications* 14 (1938): 268.

Hand, Wayland D. "'The Fear of the Gods': Superstition and Popular Belief." *American Folklore: Voice of America Forum Lectures*. Ed. Tristam Potter Coffin. Washington, D.C.: U.S. Information Service, 1968. 215–27.

——. "More Popular Beliefs and Superstitions from Pennsylvania." *Two Penny Ballads and Four Dollar Whiskey*. Ed. Robert H. Byington and Kenneth S. Goldstein. Hatboro, Penn.: Folklore Associates, 1965.

Hand, Wayland D., and Marjorie Griffin. "Inhalants in Respiratory Disorders." *Journal of American Folklore* 77 (1964): 258–61.

Hand, Wayland D., Anna Casetta, and Sondra B. Thiederman, eds. *Popular Beliefs and Superstitions: A Compendium of American Folklore from the Ohio Collection of Newbal Niles Puckett*. Boston: Hall, 1981.

Hatch, E. LeRoy. "Home Remedies Mexican Style." *Western Folklore* 28 (1969): 163–68.

Hendricks, George D. *Mirrors, Mice, and Mustaches: A Sampling of Superstitions and Popular Beliefs in Texas*. Austin: Texas Folklore Society, 1966.

——. "Superstitions Collected in Denton, Texas." *Western Folklore* 15 (1956): 1–18.

Herman, Bernard L. "Folk Medical Recipes in Nineteenth-Century American Farm Journals." *Pennsylvania Folklife* 25.4 (1976): 16–25.

Herrera, Mary A. "The Miseries and Folk Medicine." *North Carolina Folklore* 20 (1972): 42–46.

Hines, Donald M. "Superstitions from Oregon." *Western Folklore* 24 (1965): 7–20.

Hunter, Earl D. "Folk Remedies on Man and Beasts." *Kentucky Folklore Record* 8.3 (1962): 97–108.

Jahoda, Gustav. *The Psychology of Superstition*. London: Allen Lane, 1969.

Kether, Kenneth L. "Superstitious Pigeons, Hydrophobia, and Conventional Wisdom." *Western Folklore* 30 (1971): 1–17.

Kinely, Harold R. "The Healing Waters of Shallotte." *North Carolina Folklore Journal* 24 (1976): 107–10.

Labarbera, Michael. "An Ounce of Prevention and Grandma Tried Them All." *New York Folklore Quarterly* 20 (1964): 126–29.

Lemley, Marian. "A Lincoln County Hiccup Cure." *North Carolina Folklore Journal* 21 (1973): 31.

Lumpkin, Ben Gray, collected by Mrs. R. C. Cooke and Mrs. E. D. Hammer. "Remedies." *Tennessee Folklore Society Bulletin* 42 (1976): 65–69.

McAtee, W. L. "Home Medication in Grant County, Indiana, in the Nineties." *Midwest Folklore* 5 (1955): 213–16.

——. "Medical Lore in Grant County, Indiana, in the Nineties." *Midwest Folklore* 8 (1958): 151–53.

McDonald, Flora. "Home Remedies." *North Carolina Folklore* 4 (1956): 17–18.

McGlasson, Cleo. "Superstitions and Folk Beliefs of Overton County." *Tennessee Folklore Society Bulletin* 7 (1941): 13–27.

McKinney, Ida Mae. "Superstitions of the Missouri Ozarks." *Tennessee Folklore Society Bulletin* 18 (1952): 104–9.

Marshall, John. "The Madstone: Its Origins and Applications in Barlow, Ballard County, Kentucky." *Kentucky Folklore Record* 24 (1978): 44–48.

Martin, Roxie. "Old Remedies Collected in the Blue Ridge Mountains." *Journal of American Folklore* 60 (1947): 184–85.

Moody, Clara Moore. "Some Folk Beliefs and Superstitions." *Mississippi Folklore Register* 1 (1967): 25–33.

Moore, Velda. "Lamar County Elixirs: Some Popular Cures for the Common Cold." *Mississippi Folklore Register* 15 (1981): 103–9.

Murphree, A., and M. Barrow. "Physician Dependence, Self-Treatment Practices, and Folk Remedies in a Rural Area." *Southern Medical Journal* 63 (1970): 403–8.

Paulsen, Frank M. "A Hair of the Dog and Some Other Hangover Cures from Popular Tradition." *Journal of American Folklore* 74 (1961): 152–68.

Pope, Genevieve. "Superstitions and Beliefs of Fleming County." *Kentucky Folklore Record* 11 (1965): 41–51.

Primm, Beny J. "Poverty, Folk Remedies, and Drug Misuse Among the Black Elderly." *Black Folk Medicine: The Therapeutic Significance of Faith and Trust*. Ed. Wilbur H. Watson. New Brunswick, N.J.: Transaction, 1984. 67–70.

Radford, E., and M. A. Radford. *Encyclopaedia of Superstitions*. New York: Greenwood, 1969.

Randolph, Vance. "Folk Beliefs in the Ozark Mountains." *Journal of American Folklore* 40 (1927): 78–93.

——. *Ozark Magic and Folklore*. Toronto: Dover, 1947.

——. "Ozark Superstitions." *Journal of American Folklore* 46 (1933): 1–21.

Relihan, Catherine M. "Folk Remedies." *New York Folklore Quarterly* 3 (1947): 81.

Schneider, L. L., in association with Robert B. Stone. *Old-Fashioned Health Remedies that Work Best*. West Nyack, N.Y.: Parker, 1977.

Shalinsky, Audrey C. "Thermal Springs as Folk Curing Mechanisms." *Folklore Forum* 18 (1985): 32–58.

Simon, Gwladys Hughes. "Folk Beliefs and Customs in an Hawaiian Community." *Journal of American Folklore* 62 (1949): 294–311.

——. "Folk Beliefs from Hawaii." *Journal of American Folklore* 65 (1952): 188.

Snow, Loudell F., Shirley M. Johnson, and Harry E. Mayhew. "The Behavioral Implications of Some Old Wives' Tales." *Obstetrics and Gynecology* 51 (1978): 727–32.

Snyder, Perry A. "Remedies of the Piney Woods Pioneer." *Mississippi Folklore Register* 7 (1973): 11–14.

Sonnedecker, Glenn. "Home Medication on the American Frontier." *Veröffentlichungen d. Int. Gesellschaft f. Geschichte d. Pharmazie* n.s. 38 (1972): 253–70.

Spinks, Martha. "'Hollow-Tail': Folk Operation for a Folk Disease." *Kentucky Folklore Record* 20 (1974): 3–8.

Stuart, Jesse. "Remedies that Stand Out in Memory." *Kentucky Folklore Record* 22 (1976): 59–63.

Sugg, Toni. "Old Folk Remedies from Greene County." *North Carolina Folklore Journal* 22 (1974): 113–14.

Thesen, Karen. *Country Remedies from Pantry, Field and Garden*. New York: Harper and Row, 1979.

Thomas, Daniel Lindsay, and Lucy Blayney Thomas. *Kentucky Superstitions*. Princeton, N.J.: Princeton University Press, 1920.

Thomson, Samuel. *A Narrative of the Life and Medical Discoveries of Samuel Thomson, Containing an Account of His System of Practice and Manner of Curing*. Columbus, Ohio: Horton Howard, 1822.

Trotter, Robert T. II. "*Greta* and *Azarcon*: A Survey of Episodic Lead Poisoning from a Folk Remedy." *Human Organization* 44.1 (1985): 64–72.

Turner, Teresa. "The Human Comedy in Folk Superstitions." *Publications of the Texas Folklore Society* 13 (1937): 146–75.

Walser, Richard. "Three Folk Cures." *North Carolina Folklore Journal* 27 (1979): 67–68.

Wannan, Bill. *Folk Medicine: A Miscellany of Old Cures and Remedies, Superstitions, and Old Wives Tales Having Particular Reference to Australia and the British Isles*. Melbourne, Australia: Hill, 1970.

Wilson, Gordon. "Animal Products and Minerals in Folk Medicines in the Mammoth Cave Region." *North Carolina Folklore Journal* 16 (1968): 177–81.

——. "'Store-Bought' Remedies in the Mammoth Cave Region." *North Carolina Folklore* 16 (1968): 58–62.

——."Swallow It or Rub It on: More Mammoth Cave Remedies." *Southern Folklore Quarterly* 31 (1967): 296–303.

Woodhull, Frost. *Ranch Remedies: Man, Bird, Beast*. Austin: Texas Folklore Society, 1930.

I. Evil Eye

Elworthy, Frederick Thomas. *The Evil Eye, An Account of this Ancient and Widespread Superstition*. London: Murray, 1895.

Gifford, Edward S. "The Evil Eye in Pennsylvania Medical History." *Keystone Folklore Quarterly* 5.3 (1960): 3.

——. *The Evil Eye. Studies in the Folklore of Vision*. New York: Macmillan, 1958.

Gordon, Benjamin Lee. "The Evil Eye." *Hebrew Medical Journal* 34 (1961): 261–92.

Herzfeld, Michael. "Meaning and Morality: A Semiotic Approach to Evil Eye Accusations in a Greek Village." *American Ethnologist* 8.3 (1981): 560–74.

Jones, Louis C. "The Evil Eye Among European Americans." *Western Folklore* 10 (1951): 11–25.

Krappe, Alexander Haggerty. *Balor with the Evil Eye*. New York: Columbia University Press, 1927.

Lykiardopoulos, Amica. "The Evil Eye: Towards an Exhaustive Study." *Folklore* 92 (1981): 221–30.

McDaniel, Walton Brooks. "The Pupula Duplex and Other Tokens of an 'Evil Eye' in the Light of Opthalmology." *Classical Philology* 13 (1918): 336–46.

Maclagan, Robert Craig. *Evil Eye in the Western Highlands*. London: Nutt, 1902.

Naff, Alixa. "Belief in the Evil Eye Among the Christian Syrian-Lebanese in America." *Journal of American Folklore* 78 (1965): 46–51.

J. Burn Healing, Blood Stopping, Wart Healing, and Thrash Cures

Adams, Beverly R. "Pa Was a Wart Doctor." *Mississippi Folklore Register* 7 (1973): 98–99.

Bundy, Colleen. "A Method for Removing Warts." *Journal of American Folklore* 59 (1946): 70.

Dorson, Richard M. "Blood Stoppers." *Southern Folklore Quarterly* 7 (1947): 105–18.

Owen, Guy. "The Flim Flam Man and the Wart Cure." *Tennessee Folklore Society Bulletin* 38 (1972): 91–93.

Rayburn, Otto Ernest. "Bloodstoppers in the Ozarks." *Midwest Folklore* 4 (1954): 213–15.

Sears, Jean Sarrazin. "A Garland of Louisiana Wart Cures." *Louisiana Folklore Miscellany* 3.2 (1971): 27–33.

Severance, Kathleen. "Crosses on Iron Skillets: Thrash Cures from Black Lake Swamp." *Louisiana Studies* 9 (1970): 207–16.

Stroup, Thomas. "A Charm for Stopping Blood." *Southern Folklore Quarterly* 1 (1937): 19–20.

K. Metaphor and Ritual

Fernandez, James W. "The Performance of Ritual Metaphors." *The Social Use of Metaphor Essays on the Anthropology of Rhetoric*. Ed. J. David Sapir and Jon Christopher Crocker. Philadelphia: University of Philadelphia Press, 1977. 100–131.

Jones, Michael Owen. "Doing What, With Which, and to Whom? The Relationship of Case History Accounts to Curing." *American Folk Medicine: A Symposium*. Ed. Wayland D. Hand. Berkeley: University of California Press, 1976. 301–14.

Joralemon, Donald. "The Performing Patient in Ritual Healing." *Social Science and Medicine* 23 (1986): 841–45.

Price, Laurie. "Ecuadorian Illness Stories: Cultural Knowledge in Natural Discourse." *Cultural Models in Language and Thought*. Eds. Dorothy Holland and Naomi Quinn. Cambridge: Cambridge University Press, 1987. 313–42.

Scheff, Thomas. *Catharsis in Healing, Ritual, and Drama*. Berkeley: University of California Press, 1979.

Van der Geest, Sjaak, and Susan Reynolds White. "The Charm of Medicines: Metaphors and Metonyms." *Medical Anthropology Quarterly* 3.4 (1989): 345–67.

L. Powwow

Aurand, A. Monroe, Jr. *The Pow-Wow Book. A Treatise on the Art of "Healing by Prayer" and "Laying on of Hands," Etc., Practiced by the Pennsylvania Germans and Others, Etc*. Harrisburg: Aurand, 1929.

Byington, Robert H. "Powwowing in Pennsylvania." *Keystone Folklore Quarterly* 9.3 (1964): 111–17.

Dluge, Robert L., Jr. "My Interview With a Powwower." *Pennsylvania Folklife* 21.4 (1972): 39–45.

Hohman, John George. "The Long Hidden Friend." Ed. Carleton F. Brown. *Journal of American Folklore* 17 (1904): 89–152.

Reimensnyder, Barbara Lou. "Powwowing in Union County: A Study of Pennsylvania German Folk Medicine in Context." Unpublished Ph.D. dissertation, University of Pennsylvania, 1982.

Snellenburg, Betty. "Four Interviews with Powwowers." *Pennsylvania Folklife* 18.4 (1969): 40–45.

Westkott, Marcia. "Powwowing in Berks County." *Pennsylvania Folklife* 19.2 (1969–70): 2–9.

Yoder, Don. "Hohman and Romanus: Origins and Diffusion of the Pennsylvania German Powwow Manual." *American Folk Medicine: A Symposium*. Ed. Wayland D. Hand. Berkeley: University of California Press, 1976.

——. "Twenty Questions on Powwowing." *Pennsylvania Folklife* 15.4 (1966): 38–40.

M. Poison and Snakes

Hand, Wayland D. "The Mole in Folk Medicine: A Survey from Indic Antiquity to Modern America II." *American Folk Medicine: A Symposium*. Ed. Wayland D. Hand. Berkeley: University of California Press, 1976.

Hertzog, Phares H. "Snakelore in Pennsylvania German Folk Medicine." *Pennsylvania Folklife* 17.2 (1967–68): 24–25.

——. "Snakes and Snakelore of Pennsylvania." *Pennsylvania Folklife* 17.1 (1967): 14–17; 17.2 (1967–68): 24–26.

Pound, Louise. "Nebraska Snake Lore." *Southern Folklore Quarterly* 10 (1946): 163–76.

Shillingsburg, Miriam J. "Virtue Enough to Cure so Venomous a Bite." *North Carolina Folklore Journal* 31 (1983): 31–37.

Sturtevant, William Curtis. "Animals and Disease in Indian Belief." *Indians, Animals and the Fur Trade: A Critique of Keepers of the Game*. Ed. Shepard Krech, III. Athens: University of Georgia Press, 1981. 177–88.

2. Popular Culture Beliefs and Practices

A. Osteopathy

Albrecht, Gary L., and Judith A. Levy. "The Professionalization of Osteopathy: Adaptation in the Medical Marketplace." *Research in the Sociology of Health Care* 2 (1982): 161–206.

Baer, Hans A. "The Reorganization and Rejuvenation of Osteopathy." *Social Science and Medicine* 15A (1981): 701–11.

Berson, Duera. *Pain Free Arthritis*. New York: Simon and Schuster, 1978.

Booth, E. R. *History of Osteopathy and Twentieth-Century Medical Practice*. Cincinnati, Ohio: Caxton, 1924.

Gevitz, Norman. *The D. O.'s: Osteopathic Medicine in America*. Baltimore: Johns Hopkins University Press, 1982.

Gevitz, Norman. "Osteopathic Medicine: From Deviance to Difference." *Other Healers: Unorthodox Medicine in America*. Ed. Norman Gevitz. Baltimore: Johns Hopkins University Press, 1988. 124–56.

Gray, Dennis. "'Arthritis: Variations in Beliefs About Joint Disease." *Medical Anthropology* 7.4 (1983): 29–46.

B. Chiropractic

Altman, N. *Chiropractice Alternative: A Spine Owner's Guide*. Los Angeles: Tarcher, 1981.

Anderson, Robert T. "Medicine, Chiropractic and Caste." *Anthropological Quarterly* 54.3 (1981): 157–65.

Cowie, James B., and Julian Roebuck. *An Ethnography of a Chiropractic Clinic: Definitions of a Deviant Situation*. New York: Free Press, 1975.

Gibbons, R. W. "Chiropractic in America: The Historical Conflicts of Cultism and Science." *Journal of Popular Culture* 10 (1977): 720–31.

Haldeman, S., ed. *Modern Developments in the Principles and Practice of Chiropractic*. New York: Appleton, 1980.

Kelner, Merrijoy, Oswald Hall, and Ian Coulter. *Chiropractors, Do They Help? A Study of Their Education and Practice*. Toronto: Fitzhenry, 1980.

Wardwell, Walter I. "Chiropractors: Evolution to Acceptance." *Other Healers: Unorthodox Medicine in America*. Ed. Norman Gevitz. Baltimore: Johns Hopkins University Press, 1988. 157–91.

——. "The Future of Chiropractic." *New England Journal of Medicine* 302 (1980): 688–90.

C. Homeopathic

Bhardwaj, S. M. "Medical Pluralism and Homeopathy: A Geographic Perspective." *Social Science and Medicine* 14B (1980): 209–16.

Coulter, Harris L. "Homeopathic Medicine." *Health for the Whole Person: The Complete Guide to Holistic Medicine*. Ed. Arthur C. Hastings, James Fadiman, and James S. Gordon. Boulder, Colo.: Westview, 1980. 395–400.

——. "Homeopathy." *Alternative Medicines: Popular and Policy Perspectives*. Ed. J. Warren Salmon. New York: Tavistock, 1984. 57–95.

Crellin, J. K. "Should Homeopathy Be Considered?" *North Carolina Medical Journal* 48.9 (1987): 447–50.

Kaufman, Martin. *Homeopathy in America: The Rise and Fall of a Medical Heresy*. Baltimore: Johns Hopkins University Press, 1972.

Wardwell, Walter I. "Orthodoxy and Heterdoxy in Medical Practice." *Social Science and Medicine* 6 (1972): 759–63.

D. Holistic

Berlinger, H. S., and J. W. Salmon. "The Holistic Alternative to Scientific Medicine: History and Analysis." *International Journal of Health Services* 10 (1980): 133–47.

Hastings, Arthur C., James Fadiman, and James S. Gordon. *Health Care for the Whole Person*. Boulder, Colo.: Westview, 1980.

Jarvis, Deforest Clinton. *Arthritis and Folk Medicine*. New York: Holt, 1960.

Kaslof, L. J., ed. *Wholistic Dimensions in Healing. A Resource Guide*. New York: Doubleday, 1978.

Malony, H. Newton. *Wholeness and Holiness: Readings in the Psychology/Theology of Mental Health*. Grand Rapids, Mich.: Baker, 1983.

Salmon, J. Warren, ed. *Alternative Medicines: Popular and Policy Perspectives*. New York: Tavistock, 1984.

Simons, Victoria. "Chiropractic." *Health for the Whole Person: The Complete Guide to Holistic Medicine*. Ed. Arthur C. Hastings, James Fadiman, and James S. Gordon. Boulder, Colo.: Westview, 1980. 227–35.

Stanway, Andrew. *Alternative Medicine: A Guide to Natural Therapies*. London: MacDonald's, 1980.

E. Biofeedback

Birk, Lee. *Biofeedback: Behavioral Medicine*. New York: Grune and Stratton, 1973.

Stoyva, Johann, et al. *Biofeedback and Self Control 1971*. Chicago: Aldine, 1972.

3. American Folk Medicine: Regional Variations

A. Southwestern

Anderson, John Q. "Texas and Southwest Medical Lore in the Anderson Collection, University of Houston." *American Folk Medicine: A Symposium*. Ed. Wayland D. Hand. Berkeley: University of California Press, 1976. 315–20.

——. *Texas Folk Medicine: 1333 Cures, Remedies, Preventives, and Health Practices*. Austin, Tex.: Encino, 1970.

Baylor, Dorothy J. "Folklore from Socorro, New Mexico." *Hoosier Folklore* 6 (1947): 149.

Black, Donald Chain. "Therapeutics for the Smiling' Mighty Jesus: Understanding East Texas Lower Class Patients' Medically Significant Departures from Standard English." *Mid-America Folklore* 8.3 (1980): 101–12.

Cowser, R. L., Jr. "Southern Folk Medicine: Texas Style." *Mississippi Folklore Register* 15 (1981): 71–83.

Martin, Harry W., et al. "Folk Illnesses Reported to Physicians in the Lower Rio Grande Valley: A Binational Comparison." *Ethnology* 24.3 (1985): 229–36.

Quebbeman, Frances E. *Medicine in Territorial Arizona*. Phoenix: Arizona Historical Foundation, 1966.

Spicer, Edward H., ed. *Ethnic Medicine in the Southwest*. Tucson: University of Arizona Press, 1977.

Trotter, Robert T., II. "Folk Medicine in the Southwest: Myths and Medical Facts." *Postgraduate Medicine* 78.8 (1985): 167–79.

B. Northeastern

Best, Martha S. "Eastern Customs of the LeHigh Valley." *Pennsylvania Folklife* 17 (1968): 2–13.

Bryan, William J. "Folk Medicine in Butler County, Pennsylvania." *Pennsylvania Folklife* 17.4 (1968): 40–43.

Crandall, F. W., and Lois Gannett. "Folk Cures of New York State." *New York Folklore Quarterly* 1 (1945): 178–80.

Cutting, Edith E. *Lore of an Adirondack County*. Ithaca, N.Y.: Cornell University Press, 1944.

Gardner, Emelyn Elizabeth. *Folklore from the Hills of Schoharie County, New York State*. Ann Arbor: University of Michigan Press, 1937.

Levine, H. D. "Folk Medicine in New Hampshire." *New England Journal of Medicine* 224.12 (1941): 487–92.

C. Southern

Barker, Catherine S. *Yesterday Today: Life in the Ozarks*. Caldwell, Idaho: Caxton, 1941.

Barrick, Mac E. "Folk Medicine in Cumberland County." *Keystone Folklore Quarterly* 9 (1964): 100–110.

Betts, Leonidas J. "Folk Medicine in Harnett County." *North Carolina Folklore Journal* 22 (1974): 84–94.

Brandon, Elizabeth. "'Traiteurs' or Folk Doctors in Southwest Louisiana." *Buying the Wind*. Ed. Richard M. Dorson. Chicago: University of Chicago Press, 1964. 261–66.

Broadfoot, Lennis Leonard. *Pioneers of the Ozarks*. Caldwell, Idaho: Caxton, 1944.

Carey, George. *Maryland Folklore and Folklife*. Cambridge, Md.: Tidewater, 1970.

Cross, Tom Peete. "Folklore from the Southern States." *Journal of American Folklore* 22 (1909): 251–55.

Green, Edward C. "A Modern Appalachian Folk Healer." *Appalachian Journal* 6.1 (1978): 2–15.

Hall, Ella R. "A Comparison of Selected Mississippi and North Carolina Remedies." *Mississippi Folklore Register* 4 (1971): 94–113.

Harrison, Lowell H. "The Folklore of Some Kentucky Slaves." *Kentucky Folklore Record* 17 (1971): 25–30.

Miller, Shari, and Miriam Rich. "Traditional Medicines." *Louisiana Folklife* 8.1 (1983): 18–19.

Musick, Ruth Ann. "West Virginia Folklore." *Hoosier Folklore* 7 (1948): 7–14.

Parker, Haywood. "Folk-Lore of the North Carolina Mountaineers." *Journal of American Folklore* 20 (1907): 241–50.

Parr, Jerry S. "Folk Cures of Middle Tennessee." *Tennessee Folklore Society Bulletin* 28 (1962): 8–12.

Porter, J. Hampden. "Notes on the Folk-Lore of the Mountain Whites of the Alleghanies." *Journal of American Folklore* 7 (1894): 105–17.

Price, Sadie F. "Kentucky Folk-Lore." *Journal of American Folklore* 9 (1901): 30–38.

Randolph, Vance. *The Ozarks: An American Survival of Primitive Society*. New York: Vanguard, 1931.

Rayburn, Otto Ernest. "The 'Granny-Woman' in the Ozarks." *Midwest Folklore* 9 (1959): 145–48.

Roberts, Leonard W., ed. "Floyd County Folklore." *Kentucky Folklore Record* 2 (1956): 33–66.

Rogers, Eliza Guy. *Early Folk Medical Practices in Tennessee*. Murfreesboro, Tenn.: Mid-South, 1941.

Shelley, Karen, and Raymond Evans. "Women Folk Healers of Appalachia." *Appalachia/America: Proceedings of the 1980 Appalachian Studies Conference*. Ed. Wilson Sommerville. Johnson City, Tenn.: Appalachian Consortium, 1981. 209–17.

Somers, J. E. "Folk Medicine in an Isolated Modern Community." *North Carolina Medical Journal* 22 (1961): 611–15.

Stekert, Ellen J. "Focus for Conflict: Southern Mountain Medical Beliefs in Detroit." *Journal of American Folklore* 83 (1970): 115–56.

Walker, John. "A Sampling of Folklore from Rutherford County, North Carolina." *North Carolina Folklore* 3.2 (1955): 6–12.

Waller, T., and Gene Killian. "Georgia Folk Medicine." *Southern Folklore Quarterly* 36 (1972): 71–91.

Whitney, Annie Weston, and Carolina Canfield Bullock. *Folk-lore from Maryland*. New York: Memoirs of the American Folklore Society, 1925.

Wiltse, Henry. "In the Field of Southern Folklore." *Journal of American Folklore* 14 (1901): 205–8.

Wright, Lillian Mayfield. "Mountain Medicine." *North Carolina Folklore* 12.1 (1964): 7–12.

D. Midwestern

Allen, John W. *Legends and Lore of Southern Illinois*. Carbondale: Southern Illinois University Area Services Division, 1963.

Black, Pauline Monette. *Nebraska Folk Cures*. University of Nebraska Studies in Language, Literature, and Criticism 15. Lincoln: University of Nebraska Press, 1935.

Davenport, Gertrude C. "Folk-Cures from Kansas." *Journal of American Folklore* 2 (1898): 129–32.

Hyatt, Harry Middleton. *Folklore from Adams County, Illinois*. New York: Memoirs of the Alma Egan Hyatt Foundation, 1935.

Pickard, Madge Evelyn, and R. Carlyle Buley. *The Midwest Pioneer: His Ills, Cures and Doctors*. Crawfordsville, Ind.: Banta, 1945.

Stout, Earl J. *Folklore from Iowa*. Memoirs of the American Folklore Society 29. New York: American Folklore Society, 1936.

E. Western

Bushnell, John H. "Medical Folklore from California." *Western Folklore* 6 (1947): 273–75.

Fife, Austin E. "Pioneer Mormon Remedies." *Western Folklore* 16 (1957): 153–62.

F. Urban

Foster, James R. "Brooklyn Folklore." *New York Folklore Quarterly* 13 (1957): 83–91.

Maloof, Patricia S. "Fieldwork and the Folk Health Sector in the Washington, D.C., Metropolitan Area." *Anthropological Quarterly* 54.2 (1981): 68–75.

Pocius, Gerald L. "Urban Folk Medicine: Some Thoughts." *Medicine et Religion Populaires/Folk Medicine and Religion*. Ed. Pierre Crepeau. Ottawa: National Museums of Canada, 1985. 113–18.

Tilney, Philip. "Some Aspects of Popular Urban Medicine." *Medicine et Religion Populaires/Folk Medicine and Religion*. Ed. Pierre Crepeau. Ottawa: National Museums of Canada, 1985. 91–100.

4. Ethnomedical Traditions in the United States

A. Native American

Beauchamp, W. "The Good Hunter and the Iroquoi Medicine." *Journal of American Folklore* 14 (1901): 153–59.

Boas, Franz. "Current Beliefs of the Kwakiutl Indians." *Journal of American Folklore* 45 (1932): 177–260.

Bourke, John G. *Medicine Men of the Apache*. Ninth Annual Report of the Bureau of Ethnology. Washington, 1892.

Corlett, William Thomas. *The Medicine Man of the American Indian and His Cultural Background*. Springfield, Ill.: Thomas, 1935.

Dixon, Mim, and Scott Kirchner. "'Poking': An Eskimo Medical Practice in Northwest Alaska." *Etudes Inuit Studies* 6.2 (1982): 109–25.

Dorsey, George. "Legend of the Teton Sioux Medicine Pipe." *Journal of American Folklore* 19 (1906): 326–29.

Ford, Richard I. "Communication Networks and Information Hierarchies in Native American Folk Medicine: Tewa Pueblos, New Mexico." *American Folk Medicine: A Symposium*. Ed. Wayland D. Hand. Berkeley: University of California Press, 1976. 143–58.

Greenlee, Robert F. "Medicine and Curing Practices of the Modern Florida Seminoles." *American Anthropologist* 46 (1944): 317–28.

Henderson, J. Neil, and Kedar K. Adour. "Comanche Ghost Sickness: A Biocultural Perspective." *Medical Anthropology* 5.2 (1981): 195–205.

Hoffman, Walter J. "The Midewiwin or 'Grand Medicine Society' of the Ojibwa." *Seventh Annual Report of the Bureau of American Ethnology 1885–1886*. Washington, D.C.: GPO, 1891.

Hrdlička, Aleš. *Physiological and Medical Observations Among the Indians of the Southwestern United States and Northern Mexico*. Bureau of American Ethnology Bulletin no. 34. Washington, D.C.: GPO, 1908.

Hudson, Charles M. *The Southeastern Indians*. Knoxville: University of Tennessee Press, 1976.

Hunter, John Dunn. *Manners and Customs of Several Indian Tribes Located West of the Mississippi*. Philadelphia: J. Maxwell, 1823. Minneapolis: Ross and Haines, 1957.

Johnson, Frank Roy. *The Tuscaroras: Mythology, Medicine, Culture*. Murfreesboro, N.C.: Johnson, 1967.

Jones, David E. *Sanapia: Comanche Medicine Woman*. New York: Holt, 1972.

MacLeish, K. "Notes of Folk Medicine in the Hopi Village of Moenkopi." *Journal of American Folklore* 56 (1943): 62–68.

Mellinger, Marie B. "The Spirit Is Strong in the Root." *Appalachian Journal* 4 (1977): 242–53.

Morgan, Lewis Henry. *League of the Ho-de-no-sau-nee or Iroquois*. 2 vols. New Haven, Conn.: Human Relations Area Files, 1954.

Parsons, Elsie Clews. "Folk-Lore of the Cherokee of Robeson County, North Carolina." *Journal of American Folklore* 32 (1919): 384–93.

Radin, Paul. *The Winnebago Tribe*. Lincoln: University of Nebraska Press, 1971.

Sandner, Donald F. "Navaho Indian Medicine and Medicine Men." *Ways of Health: Holistic Approaches to Ancient and Contemporary Medicine*. Ed. David S. Sobel. New York: Harcourt Brace Jovanovich, 1979. 117–46.

Stefánsson, V. "Notes on the Theory and Treatment of Diseases Among the Mackenzie River Eskimo." *Journal of American Folklore* 93 (1908): 43–45.

Tantaquidgeon, Gladys. "Folk Medicine of the Delaware and Related Algonkian Indians." *Anthropological Series* 3. Harrisburg: Pennsylvania Historical and Museum Commission, 1972.

Vogel, Virgil J. "American Indian Foods Used as Medicine." *American Folk Medicine: A Symposium*. Ed. Wayland D. Hand. Berkeley: University of California Press, 1976. 125–41.

Wallis, W. D. "Medicines Used by the Micmac Indians." *American Anthropologist* 24 (1922): 24–30.

Welch, Charles E., Jr. "Some Drugs of the North American Indian—Then and Now." *Keystone Folklore Quarterly* 9 (1964): 83–99.

B. African-American

Blake, J. Herman. "'Doctor Can't Do Me No Good': Social Concomitants of Health Care Attitudes and Practices Among Elderly Blacks in Isolated Rural Populations." *Black Folk Medicine: The Therapeutic Significance of Faith and Trust*. Ed. Wilbur H. Watson. New Brunswick, N.J.: Transaction, 1984. 33–40.

Brewer, John Mason. *American Negro Folklore*. Chicago: Quadrangle, 1968.

Dougherty, Molly C. *Becoming a Woman in Rural Black Culture*. New York: Holt, 1982.

Herskovits, Melville J. *The Myth of the Negro Past*. New York: Peter Smith, 1941.

Hill, Carole E. "Black Healing Practices in the Rural South." *Journal of Popular Culture* 6 (1973): 849–53.

Hurston, Zora Neale. *Mules and Men*. Bloomington: Indiana University Press, 1935.

Jackson, Jacquelyne Johnson. "Urban Black Americans." *Ethnicity and Medical Care*. Ed. Alan Harwood. Cambridge, Mass.: Harvard University Press, 1981. 37–129.

Rich, Carroll. "Born with the Veil: Black Folklore in Louisiana." *Journal of American Folklore* 85 (1976): 328–31.

Scott, Patricia Bell. "Black Folklore in Tennessee: A Working Bibliography." *Tennessee Folklore Society Bulletin* 44 (1978): 130–33.

Sims, Barbara B. "Facts in the Life History of a Black Mississippi-Louisiana Healer." *Mississippi Folklore Register* 15 (1981): 63–70.

Steward, Horace. "Kindling Hope in the Disadvantaged: A Study of the Afro-American Healer." *Mental Hygiene* 55 (1971): 96–100.

Watson, Wilbur H. "Folk Medicine and Older Blacks in Southern United States." *Black Folk Medicine: The Therapeutic Significance of Faith and Trust*. Ed. Wilbur H. Watson. New Brunswick, N.J.: Transaction, 1984. 53–66.

Watson, Wilbur H., ed. *Black Folk Medicine: The Therapeutic Significance of Faith and Trust*. New Brunswick, N.J.: Transaction, 1984.

C. Hispanic

Baca, Josephine E. "Some Health Beliefs of the Spanish Speaking." *American Journal of Nursing* 69 (1969): 2172–74.

Clark, M. Margaret. *Health in the Mexican-American Culture: A Community Study*. Berkeley: University of California Press, 1959.

Foster, George M. "Relationships Between Spanish and Spanish-American Folk Medicine." *Journal of American Folklore* 66 (1953): 201–17.

Graham, Joe S. "Folk Medicine and Intracultural Diversity Among West Texas Mexican Americans." *Western Folklore* 44 (1985): 168–93.

———. "The Role of the Curandero in the Mexican American Folk Medicine System in West Texas." *American Folk Medicine: A Symposium*. Ed. Wayland D. Hand. Berkeley: University of California Press, 1976. 169–89.

Granger, Byrd Howell. "Some Aspects of Folk Medicine Among Spanish-Speaking People in Southern Arizona." *American Folk Medicine: A Symposium*. Ed. Wayland D. Hand. Berkeley: University of California Press, 1976. 191–202.

Guerra, Francisco. "Medical Folklore in Spanish America." *American Folk Medicine: A Symposium*. Ed. Wayland D. Hand. Berkeley: University of California Press, 1976. 169–74.

Harwood, Alan. "Mainland Puerto Ricans." *Ethnicity and Medical Care*. Ed. Alan Harwood. Cambridge, Mass.: Harvard University Press, 1981. 397–81.

Hauptmann, O. H. "Spanish Folklore from Tampa, Florida (No. IV): Superstitions." *Southern Folklore Quarterly* 2 (1938): 11–30.

Hudson, Wilson Mathis, ed. *The Healer of Los Olmos and Other Mexican Lore*. Dallas: Texas Folklore Society, 1951.

McCurry, Margie F., ed. *Viva La Diferencia . . . A Chicano Cultural Awareness Conference with Emphasis on Health: A Compact Review of the Conference Held at Ghost Ranch*. Abiquiu, N.M., May 14–17, 1972. Albuquerque: University of New Mexico Press, n.d.

Madsen, William. *Mexican-Americans of South Texas*. New York: Holt, 1964.

Neighbors, Keith A. "Mexican-American Folk Diseases." *Western Folklore* 28 (1969): 249–59.

Rubel, Arthur J. "Concepts of Disease in Mexican-American Culture." *American Anthropologist* 62 (1960): 795–814.

———. "The Epidemiology of a Folk Illness: 'Susto' in Hispanic America." *Ethnology* 3 (1964): 268–83.

Sandoval, Mercedes. "Santeria as a Mental Health Care System: An Historical Overview." *Social Science and Medicine* 13 B (1979): 137–51.

Scheper-Hughes, N., and D. Stewart. "Curanderismo in Taos County, New Mexico—A Possible Case of Anthropological Romanticism?" *Western Journal of Medicine* 139 (1983): 875–84.

Schreiber, Janet M., and John P. Homiak. "Mexican Americans." *Ethnicity and Medical Care*. Ed. Alan Harwood. Cambridge, Mass.: Harvard University Press, 1981. 264–336.

Trotter, Robert T., II. "Community Morbidity Patterns and Mexican American Folk Illnesses: A Comparative Methodology." *Medical Anthropology* 7.1 (1983): 33–44.

Trotter, Robert T., II, and Juan Antonio Chavira. *Curanderismo: Mexican American Folk Healing*. Athens: University of Georgia Press, 1981.

——. "Curanderismo: An Emic Theoretical Perspective of Mexican-American Folk Medicine." *Medical Anthropology* 4.4 (1980): 423–87.

Weclew, Robert V. "The Nature, Prevalence, and Level of Awareness of 'Curanderismo' and Some of Its Implications for Community Mental Health." *Community Mental Health Journal* 11 (1975): 145–54.

D. Pennsylvania-German

Brendle, Thomas R., and Claude W. Unger. *Folk Medicine of the Pennsylvania Germans: The Non-Occult Cures*. Proceedings of the Pennsylvania German Society, 45. Norristown, Pa., 1935.

Colbert, Lisa. "Amish Attitudes and Treatment of Illness." *Pennsylvania Folklife* 30.1 (1980): 9–15.

Doering, J. Frederick. "Pennsylvania-German Folk Medicine in Waterloo County, Ontario." *Journal of American Folklore* 49 (1936): 194–98.

Egeland, Janice. "Beliefs and Behavior as Related to Illness: A Community Case Study of the Old Order Amish." 2 vols. Ph.D. Dissertation, Yale University, 1967.

Hoffman, W. J. "Folk Medicine of the Pennsylvania Germans." *Proceedings of the American Philosophical Society* 26 (1889): 329–52.

Hostetler, John A. "Folk and Scientific Medicine in Amish Society." *Human Organization* 22 (1963–64): 271–75.

——. "Folk Medicine and Sympathy Healing Among the Amish." *American Folk Medicine: A Symposium*. Ed. Wayland D. Hand. Berkeley: University of California Press, 1976. 249–58.

McCorkle, Thomas, and Jocham von Heeringen. *Culture and Medical Behavior of the Old Order Amish of Johnson County, Iowa*. Mimeographed, Iowa State University of Science and Technology, Institute of Agriculture Medicine Bulletin, no. 2. Iowa City, 1958.

Starr, Frederick. "Some Pennsylvania German Lore." *Journal of American Folklore* 4 (1891): 321–26.

E. Asian-American

Anderson, James N. "Health and Illness in Philippino Immigrants." *Western Journal of Medicine* 139.6 (1983): 811–19.

Firestone, Melvin M. "Shephardic Folk Curing in Seattle." *Journal of American Folklore* 75 (1962): 301–10.

Fitzpatrick-Nietschmann, Judith. "Pacific Islanders—Migration and Health." *Western Journal of Medicine* 139.6 (1983): 848–53.

Gould-Martin, Katherine, and Chorswang Ngin. "Chinese Americans." *Ethnicity and Medical Care*. Ed. Alan Harwood. Cambridge, Mass.: Harvard University Press, 1981. 130–71.

Lock, Margaret. "Japanese Responses to Social Change—Making the Strange Familiar." *Western Journal of Medicine* 139.6 (1983): 829–34.

Moser, John. "Indochinese Refugees and American Health Care: Adaptive Comparison of

Cambodians and Hmong." *Third World Medicine and Social Change*. Ed. John H. Morgan. New York: University Press of America, 1983. 141–56.
Muecke, Marjorie A. "Caring for Southeast Asian Refugee Patients in the USA." *American Journal of Public Health* 73 (1983): 431–36.
——. "In Search of Healers—Southeast Asian Refugees in the American Health Care System." *Western Journal of Medicine* 139.6 (1983): 835–40.
Sargent, Carolyn, et al. "Tiger Bones, Fire, and Wine: Maternity Care in a Kampuchean Refugee Community." *Medical Anthropology* 7.4 (1983): 67–79.

5. Ethnomedical Traditions in the World

A. Latin American

Hill, Carole E. "Local Health Knowledge and Universal Primary Health Care: A Behavioral Case from Costa Rica." *Medical Anthropology* 9.1 (1985): 11–24.
Logan, Michael. "Humoral Medicine in Guatemala and Peasant Acceptance of Modern Medicine." *Human Organization* 32 (1973): 385–95.
Madsen, Claudia. *A Study of Change in Mexican Folk Medicine*. New Orleans: Tulane University Press, 1965.
Schendel, Gordon. *Medicine in Mexico: From Aztec Herbs to Betatrons*. Austin: University of Texas Press, 1968.
Simmons, Ozzie. "Popular and Modern Medicine in Mestizo Communities of Coastal Peru and Chile." *Journal of American Folklore* 68 (1955): 57–71.
Williams, Harvey. "Organization and Delivery of Health Care: A Study of Change in Nicaragua." *Third World Medicine and Social Change*. Ed. John H. Morgan. New York: University Press of America, 1983. 285–95.
Young, James Clay. *Medical Choice in a Mexican Village*. New Brunswick, N.J.: Rutgers University Press, 1981.

B. Caribbean

Beckwith, Martha Warren. *Black Roadways: A Study of Jamaican Folklife*. Chapel Hill: University of North Carolina Press, 1929.
Dow, J. "Primitive Medicine in Haiti." *Bulletin of the History of Medicine* 39 (1965): 34–52.
Hill, Carole E., and Lisa Cottrell. "Traditional Mental Disorders in a Developing West Indian Community in Costa Rica." *Anthropological Quarterly* 59 (1986): 1–14.
Kiev, Ari. "Folk Psychiatry in Haiti." *Journal of Nervous and Mental Diseases* 132 (1961): 260–65.
Laguerre, Michel S. *Afro-Caribbean Folk Medicine*. Granby, Mass.: Bergin and Garvey, 1987.
Mitchell, Faith N. "Popular Medical Concepts in Jamaica and Their Impact on Drug Use." *Western Journal of Medicine* 139.6 (1983): 841–47.
Scott, Clarissa S. "Health and Healing Practices among Five Ethnic Groups in Miami, Fla." *Public Health Reports* 89 (1974): 524–32.

C. African

Bryant, Alfred T. *Zulu Medicine and Medicine-Men*. Cape Town, South Africa: Struik, 1966.
Crapanzano, Vincent. *The Hamadsha: A Study in Moroccan Ethnopsychiatry*. Berkeley: University of California Press, 1973.
Edgerton, Robert B. "Conceptions of Psychosis in Four East African Societies." *American Anthropologist* 68 (1966): 408–25.

Evans-Pritchard, E. E. *Witchcraft, Oracles, and Magic among the Azande*. Oxford: Clarendon Press.

Harley, George Way. *Native African Medicine: With Special Reference to Its Practice in the Native African Tribe of Liberia*. Cambridge, Mass.: Harvard University Press, 1941.

Horton, Robin. "African Traditional Thought and Western Science." *Africa* 37 (1967): 50–71, 155–87.

Imperato, Pascal James. *African Folk Medicine: Practices and Beliefs of the Bambara and Other Peoples*. Baltimore: York, 1977.

Janzen, John M. *The Quest for Therapy in Lower Zaire*. Berkeley: University of California Press, 1978.

Messing, Simon D. "Group Therapy and Social Status in the Zar Cult of Ethiopia." *American Anthropologist* 60 (1958): 1120–26.

Ngubane, Harriet. "Aspects of Clinical Practice and Traditional Organization of Indigenous Healers in South Africa." *Social Science and Medicine* 15B (1981): 361–65.

Staugard, Frants. "Traditional Medicine in a Developing Country: A Study of the Use of Scientific Medicine and Traditional Health Care in a Rural District of Botswana." *Folk Medicine and Health Culture: Role of Folk Medicine in Modern Health Care*. Ed. Tuula Vaskilampi and Carol MacCormack. Kuopio, Finland: University of Kuopio Press, 1982. 212–34.

D. Asian

Croizier, Ralph C. *Traditional Medicine in Modern China: Science, Nationalism, and the Tensions of Cultural Change*. Cambridge, Mass.: Harvard University Press, 1968.

Leslie, Charles, ed. *Asian Medical Systems: A Comparative Study*. Berkeley: University of California Press, 1968.

Lindenbaum, Shirley. *Kuru Sorcery: Disease and Danger in the New Guinea Highlands*. Palo Alto, Calif.: Mayfield, 1979.

Lock, Margaret. *East Asian Medicine in Urban Japan: Varieties of the Medical Experience*. Berkeley: University of California Press, 1986.

Mandelbaum, David G. "Curing and Religion in South Asia." *Journal of the Indian Anthropological Society* 5 (1970): 171–86.

Marriott, McKim. "Western Medicine in a Village of Northern India." *Health, Culture, and Community*. Ed. B. D. Paul. New York: Russell Sage Foundation, 1955. 239–68.

Opler, Morris. "The Cultural Definition of Illness in Village India." *Human Organization* 22 (1963): 32–35.

Sidel, Victor W. "The Barefoot Doctors of the People's Republic of China." *New England Journal of Medicine* 286 (1972): 1292–1300.

Taylor, Carl E., et al. "Asian Medical Systems: A Symposium on the Role of Comparative Sociology in Improving Care." *Social Science and Medicine* 7 (1973): 307–18.

Udupa, K. N. "The Ayurvedic System of Medicine in India." *Health by the People*. Ed. K. W. Newell. Geneva: World Health Organization, 1975. 53–69.

Zimmer, Henry R. *Hindu Medicine*. Edited with a foreword and preface by Ludwig Edelstein. Baltimore: Johns Hopkins University Press, 1948.

E. British

Buckley, Anthony D. "Unofficial Healing in Ulster." *Ulster Folklife* 26 (1980): 15–34.

Dalyell, Sir John Graham. *The Darker Superstitions of Scotland*. Glasgow: Griffin, 1835.

Jones, Anne E. "Folk Medicine in Living Memory in Wales." *Folklife: A Journal of Ethnological Studies* 18 (1980): 58–68.

F. European

Davis, James M. "Tarantulas, Werewolves, and Mallow: Italian Folk Remedies in the United States." *Mississippi Folklore Register* 15 (1981): 85–95.

Georges, Robert A. "Greek Folk Remedy in America." *Southern Folklore Quarterly* 26 (1962): 122–26.

Kourennoff, Paul M. *Russian Folk Medicine*. Trans., ed., and arr. George St. George. London: Allen, 1970.

Pitre, Guiseppe. *Sicilian Folk Medicine*. Trans. by Phyllis H. Williams. Lawrence, Kans.: Coronado, 1971.

Scheper-Hughes, Nancy. *Saints, Scholars, and Schizophrenics: Mental Illness in Rural Ireland*. Berkeley: University of California Press, 1979.

Schmeller, Helmut J. "The Practice of Folk Medicine Among Volga Germans in Kansas." *Heritage of the Great Plains* 15.1 (1982): 11–16.

Williams, Phyllis H. *South Italian Folkways: A Handbook for Social Workers, Visiting Nurses, School Teachers, and Physicians*. New Haven, Conn.: Yale University Press, 1938.

6. History of Medicine

Black, William George. *Folk-Medicine: A Chapter in the History of Culture*. 1883. New York: Burt Franklin, 1970.

Bonser, Wilfrid. *The Medical Background of Anglo-Saxon England: A Study in History, Psychology, and Folklore*. London: Wellcome Historical Medical Library, 1963.

Brown, Maurice C. "Early Pharmaceutics in the Deep South." *Mississippi Folklore Register* 8 (1974): 232–40.

Brown, Richard D. "The Healing Arts in Colonial and Revolutionary Massachusetts: The Context for Scientific Medicine." *Medicine in Colonial Massachusetts, 1620–1820*. Ed. Philip Cash, Eric H. Christianson, and J. Worth Estes. Boston: Colonial Society of Massachusetts, 1980.

Cash, Philip, Eric H. Christianson, and J. Worth Estes, eds. *Medicine in Colonial Massachusetts, 1620–1820*. A conference held May 25–26, 1978 by the Colonial Society of Massachusetts. Boston: Colonial Society of Massachusetts, 1980.

Cassidy, Clair M., Hans Baer, and Barbara Becker. "Selected References on Professionalized Heterodox Health Systems in English-Speaking Countries." *Medical Anthropology Quarterly* 17 (1985): 10–18.

Clements, Forrest Edward. *Primitive Concepts of Disease*. Berkeley: University of California Press, 1932.

Clifford, Terry. *Cures*. New York: Macmillan, 1980.

Duffy, John, ed. *The Rudolph Matas History of Medicine in Louisiana*. Baton Rouge: Louisiana State University Press, 1962.

Estes, J. Worth. "Therapeutic Practice in Colonial New England." *Medicine in Colonial Massachusetts, 1620–1820*. Ed. Philip Cash, Eric H. Christianson, and J. Worth Estes. Boston: Colonial Society of Massachusetts, 1980. 289–380.

Gebhard, Bruno. "Historical Relationship Between Scientific and Lay Medicine for Present-Day Patient Education." *Bulletin of the History of Medicine* 32 (1957): 46–53.

Gevitz, Norman. *Other Healers: Unorthodox Medicine in America*. Baltimore: Johns Hopkins University Press, 1988.

——. "Sectarian Medicine." *Journal of the American Medical Association* 257.12 (1987): 1636–40.

Gordon, Benjamin Lee. *Medieval and Renaissance Medicine*. New York: Philosophical Library, 1959.

Lacourciere, Luc. "A Survey of Folk Medicine in French Canada from Early Times to the Present." *American Folk Medicine: A Symposium*. Ed. Wayland D. Hand. Berkeley: University of California Press, 1976. 203–14.

Nixon, P. I . *A Century of Medicine in San Antonio*. San Antonio, Tex.: privately printed, 1936.

Novotny, Ann, and Carter Smith. *Images of Healing: A Portfolio of American Medical and Pharmaceutical Practice in the 18th, 19th, and Early 20th Centuries*. New York: Macmillan, 1980.

Plinius, Secundus C. *Natural History*. Ed. T. E. Page et. al. 10 vols. Cambridge: Loeb Classical Library, 1938–62.

Puhvel, Jaan. "The Mole in Folk Medicine: A Survey from Indic Antiquity to Modern America." *American Folk Medicine: A Symposium*. Ed. Wayland D. Hand. Berkeley: University of California Press, 1976. 31–36.

Svensson, Jon-Erik. *Compendium of Early American Folk Remedies, Receipts and Advice*. New York: Berkeley, 1977.

Talbot, Charles H. "Folk Medicine and History." *American Folk Medicine: A Symposium*. Ed. Wayland D. Hand. Berkeley: University of California Press, 1976.

——. *Medicine in Medieval England*. London: Oldbourne, 1967.

7. General Studies in Medical Folklore

Aikman, Lonnelle. *Nature's Healing Arts: From Folk Medicine to Modern Drugs*. Washington, D.C.: National Geographic Society, 1977.

Black, William George. *Folk-Medicine: A Chapter in the History of Culture*. London: Folk-Lore Society, 1883.

Friedman, Daniel. "Anatomy of Ambiguous Folk Medicine." *Folk Medicine and Health Culture: Role of Folk Medicine in Modern Health Care*. Ed. Tuula Vaskilampi and Carol MacCormack. Kuopio, Finland: University of Kuopio Press, 1982. 17–27.

Gaddis, Vincent. "The Varieties of Healing Experience." *False and True Stories of the Strange and Unknown* 25 (1972): 73–80.

Gebhard, Bruno. "The Interrelationship of Scientific and Folk Medicine in the United States of America Since 1850." *American Folk Medicine: A Symposium*. Ed. Wayland D. Hand. Berkeley: University of California Press, 1976. 87–98.

Guldbeck, Per E. "A Perspective on Folk Medicine." *New York Folklore Quarterly* 18 (1962): 163–72.

Hand, Wayland D. "Comparative Folk Medicine: The New Agendum." *Folklore Forum* 16 (1983): 249–61.

——. "The Folk Healer: Calling and Endowment." *Journal of the History of Medicine and the Allied Sciences* 26 (1971): 263–75.

Heindel, Ned D., and Natalie I. Foster. "Medicine, Music, and 'Money' Munyon." *Pennsylvania Folklife* 32.1 (1982): 44–48.

Hines, Donald M. "A Finder for Folk Cures." *Southern Folklore Quarterly* 30 (1966): 301–4.

Honko, Lauri. "Folk Medicine and Health Care Systems." *Scandinavian Yearbook of Folklore* 38 (1982): 57–85.

——. "On the Effectivity of Folk-Medicine." *Arv* 18–19 (1962–63): 290–300.

Houston, W. R. "The Doctor Himself as a Therapeutic Agent." *Annals of Internal Medicine* 11 (1938): 1416–25.

Hufford, David J. "Folk Healers." *Handbook of American Folklore*. Ed. Richard M. Dorson. Bloomington: Indiana University Press, 1983. 306–13.

Jacob, Dorothy. *Cures and Curses*. New York: Taplinger, 1967.

Jarvis, Deforest Clinton. *Folk Medicine: A Vermont Doctor's Guide to Good Health*. New York: Holt, 1958.

Jones, Louis C. "Practitioners of Folk Medicine." *Bulletin of the History of Medicine* 23 (1949): 480–93.

La Barre, Weston. "Folklore and Psychology." *Journal of American Folklore* 61 (1948): 382–90.

——. "Folk Medicine and Folk Science." *Journal of American Folklore* 55 (1942): 197–203.

Meyer, Clarence. *American Folk Medicine*. New York: Crowell, 1973. Glenwood, Ill.: Meyerbooks, 1985.

Monteiro, Lois A. "Nursing Lore." *New York Folklore Quarterly* 29 (1973): 97–110.

Nations, Marilyn K., Linda A. Camino, and Frederic B. Walder. "'Hidden' Popular Illnesses in Primary Care: Residents' Recognition and Clinical Implications." *Culture, Medicine, and Psychiatry* 9 (1985): 223–40.

Pet, Loren H. "Dr. Bear's Medical Folklore." *Seattle Folklore Society Journal* (1973): 13.

Powles, John. "On the Limitations of Modern Medicine." *Science, Medicine, and Man* 1 (1973): 1–30.

Santino, Jack. "On the Nature of Healing as a Folk Event." *Western Folklore* 44 (1985): 153–67.

Schmitt, Lavonne E. "A Nurse Studies Folk Self-Care Practices." *Mississippi Folklore Register* 10 (1976): 71–88.

Shaw, Carol. "Memories of a Folk Doctor: Dr. Cicero West." *North Carolina Folklore Journal* 28 (1980): 22–41.

Shryock, Richard Harrison. *Medicine in America*. Baltimore: Johns Hopkins University Press, 1966.

Trimmer, Eric J. "Medical Folklore and Quackery." *Folklore* 75 (1965): 161–75.

Vaskilampi, Tuula, and Carol MacCormack, eds. *Folk Medicine and Health Culture: Role of Folk Medicine in Modern Health Care*. Kuopio, Finland: University of Kuopio, 1982.

Vuori, Hannu. "World Health Organization and Traditional Medicine." *Folk Medicine and Health Culture: Role of Folk Medicine in Modern Health Care*. Ed. Tuula Vaskilampi and Carol MacCormack. Kuopio, Finland: University of Kuopio Press, 1982. 165–89.

Watson, Wilbur H. "Central Tendencies in the Practice of Folk Medicine." *Black Folk Medicine: The Therapeutic Significance of Faith and Trust*. Ed. Wilbur H. Watson. New Brunswick, N.J.: Transaction, 1984. 87–97.

Wilson, Charles B. "Notes on Folk-Medicine." *Journal of American Folklore* 21 (1908): 68–73.

Wilson, Gordon, and Jesse Funk. "Folklore in Certain Professions: The Physician and the Folklore." *Tennessee Folklore Society Bulletin* 35 (1969): 1–5.

Wilson, Gordon, and Mr. and Mrs. Raymond Hazelip. "Folklore in Certain Professions: The Pharmacist and Folklore." *Tennessee Folklore Society Bulletin* 35 (1969): 113–16.

Wolf, John Quincy. "Two Folk Scientists in Action." *Tennessee Folklore Society Bulletin* 25 (1969): 6–10.

8. General Studies in Medical Anthropology

Ackerknecht, Erwin H. *Medicine and Ethnology: Selected Essays*. Baltimore: Johns Hopkins University Press, 1971.

——. *Therapeutics: From the Primitives to the Twentieth Century*. Stuttgart: Enke, 1973.

Chrisman, Noel J., and Thomas W. Maretzki, eds. *Clinically Applied Anthropology: Anthropologists in Health Science Settings*. Boston: Reidel, 1982.

Clark, M. Margaret, special guest editor. "Cross Cultural Medicine." *The Western Journal of Medicine* 139.6 (1983): 805–983.

Dubos, René Jules. *Man Adapting*. New Haven, Conn.: Yale University Press, 1965.

——. *Mirage of Health: Utopias, Progress and Biological Change*. New York: Perennial, 1971.

Fabrega, Horatio, Jr. "On the Specificity of Folk Illnesses." *Southwestern Journal of Anthropology* 26 (1970): 305–14.

Gonzalez, Nancie L. "Cultural and Environmental Factors in the Definition and Understanding of Health." *Assessing the Contributions of the Social Sciences to Health*. Ed. Harvey M. Brenner, Anne Mooney, and Thomas J. Nagy. Boulder, Colo.: Westview, 1980. 147–58.

Harwood, Alan, ed. *Ethnicity and Medical Care*. Cambridge, Mass.: Harvard University Press, 1981.

Hughes, Charles C. "Ethnomedicine." *International Encyclopedia of the Social Sciences*. Vol. 10. New York: Free Press/Macmillan, 1968.

Klein, Norman, ed. *Culture, Curers and Contagion*. Novato, Calif.: Chandler, 1979.

Kleinman, Arthur. "Indigenous and Traditional Systems of Healing." *Health for the Whole Person: The Complete Guide to Holistic Medicine*. Ed. Arthur C. Hastings, James Fadiman, and James S. Gordon. Boulder, Colo.: Westview, 1980. 427–35.

——. "Some Issues for a Comparative Study of Medical Healing." *International Journal of Social Psychiatry* 19 (1973): 159–65.

——. "Toward a Comparative Study of Medical Systems: An Integrated Approach to the Study of the Relationship of Medicine and Culture." *Science, Medicine, and Man* 1 (1973): 55–65.

Koss, Joan D. "Ethnomedicine, or Comparative Medical Systems." *Teaching Medical Anthropology: Model Courses for Graduate and Undergraduate Instruction*. Ed. Harry F. Todd, Jr., and Julio Ruffini. Washington, D.C.: Society for Medical Anthropology, 1979. 29–40.

Landy, David, ed. *Culture, Diseases, and Healing: Studies in Medical Anthropology*. New York: Macmillan, 1977.

Logan, Michael H., and Edward E. Hunt, Jr., eds. "Health and the Human Condition." *Perspectives on Medical Anthropology*. Belmont, Calif.: Wadsworth, 1978.

Moore, Lorna G., et al. *The Biocultural Basis of Health: Expanding Views of Medical Anthropology*. St. Louis, Mo.: Mosby, 1980.

Morley, Peter, and Roy Wallis, eds. *Culture and Curing: Anthropological Perspectives on Traditional Medical Beliefs and Practices*. Pittsburgh: University of Pittsburgh Press, 1979.

Nader, Laura, and Thomas W. Maretzki, eds. *Cultural Illness and Health*. Washington, D.C.: American Anthropological Association, 1973.

Polgar, S. "Health and Human Behavior: Areas of Interest Common to the Social and Medical Sciences. *Current Anthropology* 3 (1962): 159–205.

Romanucci-Ross, Lola, Daniel E. Moerman, and Laurence R. Tancredi, eds. *The Anthropology of Medicine: From Culture to Method*. New York: Praeger, 1983.

Saunders, Lyle. *Cultural Difference and Medical Care*. New York: Russell Sage Foundation, 1954.

Todd, Harry F., Jr., and Julio L. Ruffini, eds. *Teaching Medical Anthropology: Model Courses for Graduate and Undergraduate Instruction*. Washington, D.C.: Society for Medical Anthropology, 1979.

Vaskilampi, Tuula. "Culture and Folk Medicine." *Folk Medicine and Heatlh Culture: Role of Folk Medicine in Modern Health Care*. Ed. Tuula Vaskilampi and Carol MacCormack. Kuopio, Finland: University of Kuopio Press, 1982. 2–16.

Young, Allan. "The Anthropologies of Illness and Sickness." *Annual Review of Anthropology* 11 (1982): 257–85.

Zimmerman, Michael R. *Foundations of Medical Anthropology: Anatomy, Physiology, Biochemistry, Pathology in Cultural Context*. Philadelphia: Saunders, 1980.

9. General Studies in Medical Sociology

Adams, Richard N., and Arthur J. Rubel. "Sickness and Social Relations." *Social Anthropology*. Ed. Nash Manning. Austin: University of Texas Press, 1967.

Albrecht, Gary L., and Paul C. Higgins, eds. *Health, Illness and Medicine: A Reader in Medical Sociology*. Chicago: Rand McNally, 1979.

Becker, Marshall H., ed. *The Health Belief Model and Personal Health Behavior*. Thorofare, N.J.: Slack, 1974.

Eichler, Lillian. *The Customs of Mankind*. New York: Doubleday, 1924.

Hinkle, Lawrence E., Jr. "The Concept of 'Stress' in the Biological and Social Sciences." *Psychosomatic Medicine: Current Trends and Clinical Applications*. Ed. Z. J. Lipowski, Don Lipsett, and Peter Whybrow. New York: Oxford University Press, 1977. 27–42.

Rosestock, I. M. "Historical Origins of the Health Belief Model." *The Health Belief Model and Personal Health Behavior*. Ed. Marshall H. Becker. Thorofare, N.J.: Slack, 1974.

Stacey, Margaret. *The Sociology of Health and Healing*. London: Unwin Hyman, 1988.

Wolinsky, Frederic D. *The Sociology of Health: Principles, Professions, and Issues*. Boston: Little, Brown, 1980.

Contributors

Karen Baldwin is Associate Professor of English at East Carolina University and Director of the ECU Folklore Archive. She holds an M.A. in folklore and a Ph.D. in folklore-folklife (1975) from the University of Pennsylvania. As a George C. Marshall Fellow in Denmark, she studied at the University of Copenhagen and the National Open Air Museum, Frilandsmuseet. She directed the Folklore Archive at Wayne State University, and taught folklore at the University of Massachusetts-Amherst. She is a specialist in family folklore and folklore and education, and has published articles and book chapters on women's traditions, oral traditional poetry, the folklore of the deaf, and family narratives. In 1979–80 Baldwin and James Kirkland did team fieldwork in folk medicine in the eastern region of North Carolina with a research grant from East Carolina University.

Richard Blaustein (Ph.D., Folklore, Indiana University, 1975) is Director of the Center for Appalachian Studies and Services, Professor of Sociology and Anthropology at East Tennessee State University, and also Adjunct Professor of Family Medicine and Psychiatry in ETSU's James H. Quillen College of Medicine. His scholarly interests include medical folklore, revitalization movements, North American folk music, and Appalachian studies; his articles and book reviews have been published in various folklore and regional studies journals.

Linda A. Camino is a cultural and medical anthropologist who received her Ph.D. from the University of Virginia. She has held appointments at the University of Virginia School of Medicine, the Virginia Department of Mental Health, Mental Retardation and Substance Abuse Services, and the International Counseling Center in Washington, D.C. Her research interests and publications are concerned with the health and mental health of African-Americans, refugees, and immigrants, and the application of anthropological theory and methods. Currently, Camino is Research Assistant Professor of Anthropology at George Washington University, is on the board of directors of the International Counseling Center, and is a consultant to several organizations engaged in cross-cultural research and service delivery.

Edward M. Croom, Jr., is an ethnobotanist with the Research Institute of Pharmaceutical Sciences at the University of Mississippi in Oxford, Mississippi. Croom has documented traditional medicines, evaluated plants as new sources of foods, drugs, and herbicides, and directed the production of artemisinin, a plant-derived antimalarial drug for clinical trials by the World Health Organization. Current research includes the enhanced production of the plant-based cancer agent taxol and the evaluation of plant medicines as a safe, effective, and affordable health care system.

David J. Hufford is Associate Professor of Behavioral Science at the Penn State College of Medicine, located at the Milton S. Hershey Medical Center where he also is Director of the Center for Humanistic Medicine and Academic Director of the Medical Ethnography Collection. He holds adjunct appointments at the University of Pennsylvania in nursing, social gerontology, and folklore-folklife, and regularly teaches graduate courses in folk medicine and in the ethnography of belief. He received his Ph.D. in folklore-folklife in 1974 from the University of Pennsylvania, was the Pennsylvania State Folklorist, and taught at Memorial University of Newfoundland. He is Chairperson of the Committee on Cultural Heritage and Delivery of Human Services of the Pennsylvania Heritage Affairs Commission and is a member of the Minority Health Advisory Committee of the Pennsylvania State Department of Health. He is the author of numerous books and articles on belief theory and folk healing.

James Kirkland is Professor of English at East Carolina University, where he teaches folklore, American literature, and rhetoric/composition. Although he has published extensively in all three areas of specialization, he has been especially active in folk medical studies, doing cooperative research with scholars in various disciplines, conducting independent investigations of folk medical beliefs and practices in eastern North Carolina, and directing student fieldwork. Among his current research interests is the Evil Eye tradition and its manifestations in folklore, popular culture, and literature.

Peter R. Lichstein received his undergraduate and medical degrees from the University of Michigan. After completing internship and residency in internal medicine at the University of North Carolina, Chapel Hill, he was instructor and fellow in medicine and psychiatry at the University of Rochester, New York. Lichstein is currently an Associate Professor of Medicine at the East Carolina University School of Medicine. He is head of the section of general internal medicine and director of the internal medicine residency program at the University Medical Center of Eastern Carolina, Pitt County. His research interests include medical anthropology, medical ethics, and the doctor-patient relationship.

Holly F. Mathews is Associate Professor of Anthropology at East Carolina University. She has applied her theoretical interest in cognitive and psychological anthropology to the study of the organization and structure of ethnomedical beliefs, medical decisionmaking, issues in cross-cultural gerontology, social organization and sex roles, and gender ideology in the United States and Latin America. Presently, she is conducting research in eastern North Carolina on alternative health care use among the rural elderly.

Robert Sammons is currently medical director of the psychiatric center at St. Mary's Hospital in Grand Junction, Colorado. He obtained his Ph.D. in clinical psychology from the University of North Carolina at Greensboro, and his M.D. from the University of North Carolina at Chapel Hill. He completed his residency in psychiatry at the University of Virginia where he did a psychology post-doctorate in behavioral medicine, as well as a fellowship in forensic psychiatry. Sammons's current folklore interest has shifted to the Southwest as has his residence, and he currently focuses his attention on Hopi Eagle Kachina and Eagle Dances.

C. W. Sullivan III is a Professor of English and the Director of Graduate Studies in English at East Carolina University. He is the current Vice-President of the International Association for the Fantastic in the Arts and the editor of *The Children's Folklore Review.* He is the author of numerous books and articles on mythology, folklore, fantasy, and science fiction.

Index

Library of Congress Cataloging-in-Publication Data
Herbal and magical medicine : traditional healing today
/ edited by James Kirkland . . . [et al.].
Includes bibliographical references and index.
ISBN 0-8223-1208-5 (cloth). —
ISBN 0-8223-1217-4 (pbk)
1. Folk medicine—Virginia. 2. Folk medicine—North
Carolina. I. Kirkland, James, 1942–
[DNLM: 1. Medicine, Traditional—North Carolina.
2. Medicine Traditional—Virginia. WB 50 AN8 H5]
GR110.V8H47 1992
615.8'82'09755—dc20
DNLM/DLC
for Library of Congress 91-25003 CIP

www.ingramcontent.com/pod-product-compliance
Lightning Source LLC
Chambersburg PA
CBHW050349270326
41926CB00016B/3656

* 9 7 8 0 8 2 2 3 1 2 1 7 8 *